# ORTHO AND COMPLEMENTARY MEDICINE

## An Alliance for a Changing World

W.H. Kirkaldy-Willis, M.D. and A.A. Swartz, M.D.

North Atlantic Books  Berkeley, California

*Orthodox and Complementary Medicine*

Published by North Atlantic Books
P.O. Box 12327
Berkeley, California 94712

Cover and book design by Nancy Koerner

Printed in the United States of America

*Orthodox and Complementary Medicine* is sponsored by the Society for the Study of Native Arts and Sciences, a nonprofit educational corporation whose goals are to develop an educational and crosscultural perspective linking various scientific, social, and artistic fields; to nurture a holistic view of arts, sciences, humanities, and healing; and to publish and distribute literature on the relationship of mind, body, and nature.

**Library of Congress Cataloging-in-Publication Data**
    Kirkaldy-Willis, W. H.
        Orthodox and complementary medicine : an alliance for a changing world /
    by William Kirkaldy-Willis and Aubrey Swartz.
          p.    cm.
    ISBN 1-55643-355-7
    1. Alternative medicine. 2. Medicine. I. Swartz, Aubrey A. II. Title.
    R733 .K565 2000
    615.5--dc21
          00-032887

1  2  3  4  5  6  7  8  9 / 04  03  02  01

# Contents

Preface . . . . . . . . . . . . . . . . . . . . . . . . . . . . . . . . . . . . . . . . . vii

Acknowledgements . . . . . . . . . . . . . . . . . . . . . . . . . . . . . . . . ix

1. Three Thousand Years Ago . . . . . . . . . . . . . . . . . . . . . . . . 1
2. A New Approach to Health Care . . . . . . . . . . . . . . . . . . . 7
3. American Back Society . . . . . . . . . . . . . . . . . . . . . . . . . . . 17

## Orthodox and Complementary Disciplines

4. Mainstream Medicine . . . . . . . . . . . . . . . . . . . . . . . . . . . 25
5. Homeopathy . . . . . . . . . . . . . . . . . . . . . . . . . . . . . . . . . . 43
6. Chiropractic . . . . . . . . . . . . . . . . . . . . . . . . . . . . . . . . . . 51
7. Osteopathy . . . . . . . . . . . . . . . . . . . . . . . . . . . . . . . . . . . 67
8. Physical Therapy . . . . . . . . . . . . . . . . . . . . . . . . . . . . . . . 75
9. Chinese Medicine, Acupuncture, and Herbal Medicine . . . . . . 81
10. Naturopathy . . . . . . . . . . . . . . . . . . . . . . . . . . . . . . . . . . 91
11. Aromatherapy . . . . . . . . . . . . . . . . . . . . . . . . . . . . . . . . . 99
12. Miscellaneous Disciplines . . . . . . . . . . . . . . . . . . . . . . . . 103

# Other Considerations

13. The Immune System . . . . . . . . . . . . . . . . . . . . . . . . . . . . . 115
14. A Word About Cancer . . . . . . . . . . . . . . . . . . . . . . . . . . . 123
15. The Influence of the Home . . . . . . . . . . . . . . . . . . . . . . . 133
16. The Workplace . . . . . . . . . . . . . . . . . . . . . . . . . . . . . . . . 137
17. The Nurse . . . . . . . . . . . . . . . . . . . . . . . . . . . . . . . . . . . 149
18. Listening and Asking . . . . . . . . . . . . . . . . . . . . . . . . . . . . 157
19. A Place to Linger . . . . . . . . . . . . . . . . . . . . . . . . . . . . . . 165
20. Current Issues . . . . . . . . . . . . . . . . . . . . . . . . . . . . . . . . 171
21. Teaching and Learning . . . . . . . . . . . . . . . . . . . . . . . . . . 177
22. Thrusting Through the Waves . . . . . . . . . . . . . . . . . . . . . . 185
23. Tomorrow's World . . . . . . . . . . . . . . . . . . . . . . . . . . . . . 191

# Preface

We have attempted to inform the reader how much each of us came to appreciate the manner in which health care providers in many different disciplines approach the problems of prevention and treatment of musculoskeletal and other lesions. There is no doubt in our minds that many disciplines beside the orthodox ones have much to offer. If there is one message that is outstanding, it is this: that in the delivery of health care, as in many other fields of endeavor, true unity lies in diversity.

We often fail to help the patient as we should, because we fail to make a correct diagnosis. It is necessary in doing this to consider not only the physical diagnosis but also the personality of the person as a whole in the context of the home, the place of work, the interests, and the belief systems of the individual. Another cause of failure is that we do not spend sufficient time in educating the patient and his or her relatives about the nature of the illness or injury nor how to help the patient return to a state of healthy well-being.

In this short book we hope to demonstrate some of the ways in which with one discipline and another we can correct these failings, as we learn to work together to produce a more acceptable, efficient, and cost-effective approach to prevention and treatment.

—A.A.Swartz, M.D. and W.H.Kirkaldy-Willis, M.D.

# Acknowledgements

The authors wish to express their thanks to Mr. Charles Stein for much help with the work involved in writing this book; to Dr. T.N. Bernard, Jr. for help with the chapter on "A New Approach to Health Care"; to the members of the American Back Society, who have stimulated us to write this book; and last, but by no means least, to our wives for their encouragement and patience during the work of writing the manuscript.

— 1 —

# Three Thousand Years Ago

HISTORIANS TELL OF centers of healing in China, Greece, and else-where more than three thousand years ago. Chinese medicine was based on the idea of the functioning of a myriad of tiny meridians, channels that traverse the whole body, and of a large compendium of natural-ly occurring plant extracts. We'll have more to say about this in a later chapter.

In ancient Greece a number of centers for the healing arts developed in places like Delphi, Cos, Pergamum, and Epidauros. Accounts of the activities of these centers are supported by historical writings, by myths that were stories with a meaning, and by archeological explorations of the ruins of what were once magnificent temples, stadia, and amphitheatres. In the modern Western world our way of living owes so much to Greek thought and action that it influences even today the ways in which we go about the prevention of disease and its healing. There was then and should be now one healing channel, albeit expressed in a variety of dif-ferent ways. We refer to unity through diversity.

Delphi, the center of healing of the god Apollo, is reached from Athens today by a hot, dusty road, the ancient Sacred Way, which skirts the sea of the Corinthian Gulf, along which many centuries ago pilgrims trudged to celebrate the Mysteries at Eleusis, passing the island of

Salamis where Themistocles smashed the Persian fleet, along the narrow street through the village of Arachova, and down the winding road leading to Delphi. As Euripedes said, "It's a long way to Delphi." From the small town of Delphi the narrow winding road leads westward to the small fishing village of Itea by the the seaside on the Gulf.

It's not difficult to imagine the time three thousand years ago when Itea was a busy port for the anchoring of the blue-and-white-hulled ships with their high prows and scarlet sails, to discharge their scores of pilgrims who, sick and troubled in body and mind, came day after day to make their offerings and seek a cure at the Temple of Apollo, god of healing. In those far off days the easy way to come from afar across the Mediterranean or Aegean Sea was by ship to Itea. For all its hazards, to come by ship was less dangerous than to travel by road across the mountains, risking bandits and wild animals.

From the port the pilgrims, their few possessions on their backs, started to trudge inland, climbed a slight ascent in the well-worn track, and from the top entered the old Pilgrims' way, winding, white, and dusty through the dark green forest of olive trees swaying in the evening breeze, wave after wave traveling across their tops like wind blowing across a field of corn. The Crissa bluff on the left hid then, as it does today, the temple columns from view, and above it rose the great cliffs at the foot of mount Parnassus, their names Flamboyant and Roseate, the Shining Ones, lit up as though by fire by the dying sun. As they and we round the bluff the magnificent tall Athenian columns of the temple suddenly materialize, these also lit by the fire of the setting sun, as they stand above the high cliffs on which the temple was built. The Temple itself is magnificent, faced by fluted Corinthian columns, though now in ruins. Nearby, hollowed out of the mountainside, are a stadium for the games and a theatre for dramatic performances, with stone seats rising up from the stage.

Accommodation for the pilgrims was simple but adequate. It's easy to imagine the excitement of the pilgrims as they struggled, travelworn and footsore, to the night's shelter in the hostel beside the Temple precincts, this the first step in the journey to health and healing. We mortals of the twentieth century in our turn must make the effort and face the sweat, fear, danger, and the spiritual ocean that we too must navigate to reach the place of healing.

We reconstruct in our minds the ancient scene: the crowd of footsore pilgrims knocking at the precinct gate: welcomed by the janitor and handed over one by one to a waiting priest or priestess: each young, attractive attendant leading his or her charge to their small cubicle and listening carefully and at length to their tale of woe. Instructed to remove the outer clothes, the pilgrim lies down on a table of raised stone to be examined by the young priest or priestess. This done in careful detail, the therapist gives the pilgrim a thorough massage, sometimes therapeutic touch, sometimes deep massage, often causing the accustomed pleasure to the weary traveler as is done in the massage parlor today.

After receiving a bitter, relaxing draught, the patient is shown a place to sleep and given blankets against the cold mountain air, warned not to be concerned about the sacred snakes that slither near for the warmth of sleeper and covering; said by some to bring the magic healing power of the god. The priest or priestess uses hypnotic power to make suggestions for the thoughts and feelings that will surely bring healing from the subconscious mind during the hours of darkness.

Each pilgrim fit for it is roused at daybreak to swim in the clear water of the temple pool, followed by exercises shown by the attendant young priest or priestess. The fast is broken by a glass of watered wine and a few crusts of rough, home-baked bread. Breakfast over, the suppliants gather for prayer to the god in the temple auditorium. This is followed by further investigation from the therapist, instruction in lifestyle, administration of the natural herbs, garlic prominent among them, and encouragement to take part in the games and exercises. These include running, often relay races, handing on the torch from one to the next, around the track in the stadium.

After a frugal midday repast there is a time appointed for rest, each in his or her cubicle, and then further instruction, according to individual need, often with further massage and manipulation of painful muscles, joints, chest, and abdomen. The attending priests and priestesses are authoritative yet sympathetic. And so the days go by in easy sequence, sometimes accompanied by minor surgery with manipulation and stretching of stiff, shortened muscles, tendons, and joints.

For many there will be a prearranged appointment with the oracle, an attractive girl scarcely out of her teens. She sits on a golden tripod in the midst of a shallow, hot, sulphurous stream till inebriated by the fumes, at which time she prophesies for the benefit of the troubled one. She speaks in language incomprehensible to all but the senior priests, who interpret according to their own plan, matching their words, like politicians today, to what they think the patient needs to hear. They terminate what they have to say with the accustomed advice: "Know thyself; be moderate in all things." Today physicians might well add "and occasionally be prepared to moderate your moderation."

This brief synopsis reminds us that no healing can take place without considerable effort on the part of the patient, that the relation between healer and sufferer is very important, that both mind and body are intimately involved.

Equally compelling events took place later on the little island of Cos in the Aegean, off the southeastern part of Asia Minor, now Turkey. Heracles, scion of the distinguished family of Aesculapius, set up a center of healing near the harbor, no doubt for the convenience of sick people traveling by sea from far and wide. His son, Hippocrates, followed in his father's footsteps, taking his training in a school of renown in Macedonia, on the mainland in northeastern Greece. He returned to Cos after his father's death, choosing to develop his practice in this small island rather than the tempting more developed centers, such as those in Delphi and Epidauros. The compound was right next to the harbor wall. It comprised a dwelling house where the young Hippocrates lived, his widowed mother the housekeeper; a clinic with a building for examining and treating those who came for help; a room set aside for surgery; and a large hall where his brother supervised their system of exercises, which now we'd call a rehabilitation program, including a setup for traction and for manipulation.

Hippocrates had the assistance of a number of young apprentices who came to him from far and wide for teaching. Each evening, teachers and students gathered under an ancient plane tree to review the day's work and benefit from the great wisdom of their teacher. As they sat in a semicircle under the tree, Hippocrates in the center, they sipped glasses of local wine, diluted with water. From activities such as these came the Hippocratic Oath, which guides and directs healers of diverse instruction in the modern world.

In the 1930s, '40s and '50s I (WHK-W) tried to put some of Hippocrates' ideas into practice in treating patients and in teaching interns and residents. In Nairobi, surgeons, interns, residents, and African staff saw every one of 100 patients twice a week together, followed by open discussion of all concerned. In the 1960s in Saskatoon, I repeated the process for three hours once each week on orthopedic rounds, over coffee, and afterwards in the communal teaching room. We first planned the teaching program for the following week, then reviewed our research, and finally gave staff and residents the opportunity to say anything that was on their minds, no holds barred. I did not always follow the suggestions made, but I realized that it was very important that everyone had the chance of contributing to the running of the department.

Each year we had several parties, usually with drinks and something to eat. These occasions were particularly effective in the summer, at Dr. John Wedge's country home outside the city. When he was building his house, the whole of the orthopedic department spent two or three whole afternoons helping with the building, encouraged by the provision of beer and hot dogs. Dr. Wedge's grandfather, Mr. Justice Hall, said on one occasion, "There can't be much wrong with a department whose members wish to get together to build a house in their spare time."

Initially we made ward rounds on the ward, going from bed to bed as we discussed patients' problems. We soon found that this was disturbing for patients in Canada, though it was the general practice in Britain, so we abolished this practice and kept our discussion until we had left the ward or the patient had left the teaching room.

After some years in Saskatoon, quite by chance, I made contact with a local chiropractor, Dr. Gordon Potter, who put me in touch with the Canadian Memorial Chiropractic College in Toronto. The president of the college arranged for two recently qualified chiropractors to spend from six to twelve months of postgraduate training at the University Hospital in Saskatoon. They took part in weekly rounds and attended outpatient clinics in orthopedics, neurology, rheumatology, and the pain clinic. Both M.D.s and chiropractors were initially doubtful of the effectiveness of this new plan, but in fact there were never any problems, and one result after some years was the development of a multidisciplinary musculoskeletal clinic, supervised by a senior chiropractor. Chiropractors, physical therapists, exercise therapists, neurologists, neurosurgeons, and orthopedic surgeons cooperated in the work of this clinic. The ideas held by Hippocrates several thousand years ago have blossomed again in Saskatoon, a flowering that has spread more widely in recent times.

The spirit of Delphi and of Cos permeates the lecture halls, classrooms, and workshops of the American Back Society, where health care professionals from all disciplines come together to learn from each other in an atmosphere of intellectual honesty and congeniality. The ultimate goal of this invigorating process is to alleviate the pain and suffering of patients with diseases and injuries affecting the neck and back. The Society's headquarters occupies a converted convent, wherein the spirit of the departed clergy permeates the corridors of this grand structure. The original brick, the belfry, and the rooftop crucifix remain, a century after it was built.

In my own practice (A. A. Swartz) of orthopedics I share the space with the American Back Society. My patients receive the benefit of interdisciplinary consultation and treatment. They are referred to those disciplines that I feel would be most appropriate for a particular patient. The eternal lamps of Apollo, Aesculapius, Heracles, and Hippocrates remain with us.

# — 2 —

# A New Approach to Health Care

IN ORDER TO UNDERSTAND how best we can approach the question of the relationship between orthodox (mainstream) and complementary (alternative) medicine, we need to refresh our memories of the nature of our world. This is best seen as a combination of Newtonian and quantum physics. Some readers will wish to read the whole chapter now. Others will wish to learn only the practical findings from quantum theory. These are listed in the resume below and in abbreviated form at the end of the chapter.

It is helpful to mention the main points now. (1) Though much medical work is definite and well defined, much is vague and uncertain. (2) There is more than one way of looking at a problem. (3) The doctor and the patient interact in the best interest of a favorable outcome. (4) There is a universal togetherness and interconnectedness among all those involved in any problem, medical or other. (5) It is the task of the doctor to treat the whole patient, a combination of mind and body. (6) Chaos theory tells us that very minor changes at the start can result in major changes at the end of a situation. (7) We call changes that lead to ill health "little ripples" and those that result in healing "little nudges." It is by using these that we can prevent and heal disease. Nudges, which are listed and discussed later in this chapter, are powerful, and we employ them frequently.

Each time of crisis is, among other things, a time for progress. Today we face a time of crisis for health care. Patients are often dissatisfied, largely because of long waiting lists and lack of adequate attention from the doctor when one does get to see him or her. Doctors are dissatisfied because they have too much to do, not enough time to give to each patient, too little financial reward, and too many regulations from governments and paying agencies. Governments are displeased because of the ever-increasing demands from both patients and doctors. Payers are on edge because of the escalation of the costs of medical care. The current low rate of reimbursement makes it difficult for the doctor to spend as much time as he or she would like with each patient. There is dissatisfaction on all sides. Each new technological advance, and there are many, adds to the cost of health care, placing an increasing financial strain on hospitals and other similar institutions. This is the extent of the crisis.

The solution, if there is one, must lie in more effective diagnosis and treatment, combined with measures that present less strain and tension for the physician, and for the patient the satisfaction of feeling that he or she is given adequate attention by a caregiver who is really interested in and anxious to help him or her, as a person with the hopes and fears common to all of us. All of these problems contribute to patient dissatisfaction and their quest for alternative methods of health care. Orthodox medicine is in essence composed of several fields, of which many are complementary.

The most reliable guide is provided by the science, and, yes, the art of physics. The old physics, of which Newton was one of the chief proponents four hundred years ago, has been brought up to date by the addition of the new physics, generally referred to as quantum mechanics. From quantum theory we learn that physical reality is both "idea-like" and "matter-like," a combination of the two. Newtonian/quantum physics looks out on a world of "stuff" with an "idea-like" aspect. If quantum mechanics is correct, there is no substantive physical world "way out there" apart from our observation of and participation with it! Rather a shock!

Physicists, particularly of the quantum breed, are people who want to find out what the world and universe are like: how they work, what exactly we are doing in them, where they and we are going. Those are very much the questions that a physician asks him or herself. That's not inappropriate, for originally the physician was a person who used physics as a foundation for his work, and in the course of doing this gave his patients one or another kind of "physic," the old name for a drug. We can consider physics as the mother-science, dealing as it does with structure and with function that's dependent on structure. The first daughter, chemistry, tells us about the formation of the nucleic acids and nucleoproteins, among other things. The second daughter, biology, tells us about the source of life, coming by means of the double helix of DNA, which again is chemistry! Only this time we call it biochemistry.

Forearmed with this knowledge, we can go ahead together to consider what the universe and our world in it are like and their relationship to orthodox, alternative, and complementary medicine.

# Orthodox, Alternative, and Complementary Medicine

There is rapidly increasing recognition on the part of those in orthodox medicine that they cannot any longer afford to disregard the claims of others in alternative and complementary medicine, who for their part are increasingly ready to cooperate. There is reason to hope that a new era is about to dawn in which, through our working together, the prevention and treatment of disease will be both much more effective and equally cost effective.

Following the old approach, the Newtonian scientist employs reductionist methods, tracing the diverse disciplines of healing back to a common source, striving from that point to move forward again to consider the holistic relationships between one and another form of medicine. The quantum approach, as we shall see later, starts at the place where all are one, closely interrelated, and from that point provides room for each type of medicine to develop as an integral part of the whole. Bell's Theorem, to be considered shortly, stresses the essential togetherness, oneness, and interrelatedness of the whole universe, our approach to medicine included. In this view, no doubt to the surprise of many and the delight of some, orthodox, alternative, and complementary forms of medicine are all one. They represent unity through diversity.

Until the early years of this century physics was Newtonian in nature—well defined, clear-cut, mechanical, like clockwork. Now, following the work of Planck and Einstein, the new physics, quantum in nature, is indeterminate, fuzzy, and cloudlike. The term "quantum" comes from the discovery made by these two brilliant men that energy, mass, and light all come in small packets—quanta. The nature of our world and of the universe is in fact a combination of the Newtonian and the quantum. We cannot ever say that one particular problem is entirely clear-cut and definite while another is fuzzy and confusing. Almost without exception every problem presented by the sick person is in part Newtonian and in part quantum.

In simple terms, we are confronted in every case by the definite and clearly determined, which we designate by the term "clocks," simply because we are dealing with a situation that is clocklike. We are also confronted by the fuzzy and indefinite, which we designate by the term "cloudlike," because it is ill-defined. We set out to try to solve the problem of the sick or injured person in terms of these "clocks" and "clouds."

---

### The Nature of the Universe and Our World
#### (Studied by Two Disciplines)

| | |
|---|---|
| **Newtonian Physics:** | **Clocks** |
| **Quantum Mechanics:** | **Clouds** |

---

The initial work done by Max Planck and Albert Einstein was the result of painstaking, scientific, laboratory work combined with intuition and interpreted by mathematics. Their discoveries have been extended over the past ninety years by the work of many physicists. Their first experiments were in the subatomic realm and once again were interpreted by the language of mathematics. Here are some of the discoveries that the new physicists have made:

**Indeterminacy.** The behavior of subatomic particles is indeterminate. Radioactivity, the decay of atomic particles, is random and unpredictable. Large numbers of such particles together follow the laws of statistics, but the exact moment of decay of individual particles is unpredictable. We can assess the rate at which this decay takes place but not which individual atoms are next in line to decay. This is atomic uncertainty. Electrons do not follow a well-defined trajectory. One moment an electron is here, the next there, with no indication how it got there. Taking the TV screen as an example, we see that the majority of electrons leaving the cathode tube at the back of the monitor travel to the right place on the screen to make the picture, but not all of them reach the right place. It isn't possible to foretell which electrons will hit the right spot and which will not. Their behaviour is unpredictable. The situation is one of fuzziness.

**Uncertainty.** The above statements give rise to the Principle of Uncertainty and Probability described by Heisenberg. He said that an observer can't determine both the position and the momentum of a sub-atomic particle at the same time. He has to choose one or other of these. In quantum mechanics the experimenter is dealing with possibilities and probabilities rather than with certainties.

**Complementarity.** Over many years scientists have described the nature of light as being sometimes in terms of waves and sometimes of particles. We now know that the result depends on the experimenter and the type of experiment set up, but how can something be both a wave and a particle? When you look for waves, that's what you'll find. When you look for particles, quanta, that's what you'll find. It all depends on the type of experiment. This we call complementarity. It applies to energy and mass too, which can be detected in particle or in wave form.

**The Observer and the observed.** The behavior of, say, an individual electron in an experimental setting depends on the presence of the experimenter, the observer. Until the observer looks at the recording apparatus to see what's happened, the electron is, we say, a ghost, in limbo. Its spin is, in scientific terms, virtually both "up" and "down." The act of observation crystallizes the matter, and the electron's spin becomes either up or down. This we call the phenomenon of "the observer and the observed." It is somewhat of a mystery that the nature of things in the world outside of us depends upon the observations of the experimenter.

***Bell's Theorem.*** The British physicist John Bell, of CERN in Switzerland, formulated what is now known as Bell's Theorem. It states that when two electrons or other particles have been in contact and then are separated, say to the distance of the moon from the earth, they will always continue to affect each other. A change in the spin of one electron will immediately, faster than the speed of light, produce the opposite spin in the other. It's as though each one is conscious of what the other is doing. There is an unexplained interconnectedness between them. In the world of men and women and their daily lives, this theorem becomes easier to grasp as we realize that we are all connected with one another. All professionals involved in the care of a patient, and the patient too, can affect one another.

***Mind and Body.*** Then there's another important discovery dealing with mind and body. It was the French philosopher Rene Descartes, in the fifteenth century, who postulated that mind and body were separate entities. The individual, he said, was composed of these two separate parts. Body could influence mind, but mind could not influence the body. This dualism has influenced our thinking and set us back for more than four hundred years. Today most theologians and scientists, including quantum physicists, believe that each person has a mental and a physical component that exist in combination, each influencing the other. We can call this one entity made of two parts.

No one of us understands this phenomenon of mind and matter. This shouldn't surprise us, for we have already seen that reality is both idealike (of the spirit) and matterlike (physical). We can say that acceptance without proof is characteristic of religion, and rejection without proof characteristic of science. As scientists we look for proof, but this is not always possible. Religion is a matter of the heart, and science, a matter of the mind. One cannot exist without the other. Mind and heart are different aspects of one individual. As scientists we look for proof. But what is proof? It is no more than playing by the rules, and who makes the rules? We do!

For the new reader it's simpler to express this last section in another way. The discovery of quantum theory was made as a number of separate items, in different experiments, on different occasions, introduced, as it were, "chunk by chunk." The first chunk of information is that light and energy can be detected as particles (quanta), and the next chunk is that subatomic particles behave in an unpredictable and indeterminate way (the TV screen, for example). The third chunk informs us that light can be detected as particles or as waves, depending on the way the experiment is set up. The next chunk, Heisenberg's Uncertainty Principle, states that one cannot determine both the location and the movement of a particle at the same time. The fifth chunk tells us that the observer and what he or she observes form an inseparable unity. The next chunk is Bell's Theorem of Interconnectedness. The last chunk defines the oneness of mind and body.

Quantum physicists admitted that they could not understand the theory they had unearthed. Nils Bohr, the Danish scientist, said that no one really understood the theory! Quantum mechanics makes sense simply because of the practical technological advances resulting from the theory (in other words, what the "chunks" teach us). Year by year new chunks are discovered. There's no end to it. And each new theoretical chunk introduces a new technological invention.

---

### Characteristics of Subatomic Particles
Energy and Light as Particles
Indeterminacy and Unpredictability
Uncertainty and Probability
Light: Waves or Particles, Complementary
Close Connection of Observer and Observed
Bell's Theorem—Interconnectedness
Oneness of Mind and Body
### Quantum Theory Applies To
The Subatomic Realm • Our Human Level
The Cosmic Universe

---

Initially it was thought that quantum mechanics applied to the sub-atomic realm only. We now know it applies equally to the macroscopic and astrophysical spheres. We shall meet the factors listed above again and again in our pursuit of the causes of failure of sick and injured people to get well again and back on the job.

It is because of the practical applications, techniques, and methods that are now available to us from quantum theory that we accept it, even though the experts who work in this field do not fully understand it. This applies to many situations in life where we do not understand the theory but accept it because it works. In practical terms this hotchpotch of quantum findings makes sense because of the technological advances that have stemmed from it. From quantum come the laser, the transistor, the electron microscope, the computer, the superconductor, our knowledge of chemical bonding and of the structure of the atom, and nuclear power. We are on the spot. We're compelled to accept the incomprehensible, because quantum theory works in practice. As scientists we look for proof, but proof is not always possible. How many people understand how an internal combustion engine, fuel cell, TV set, or refrigerator function? Our ignorance doesn't worry us when we're dealing with things of practical use.

Our minds work partly by logic and partly by intuition. We accept the help of a chiropractor, osteopath, or physical therapist when suffering from neck and arm pain after too prolonged a session at the computer, because we know from experience that one or another of them can help us in a simple yet satisfactory way, whether we understand it or not.

---

**Practical Quantum Technologies**
**The Laser     The Transistor**
**Electron Microscope     Superconductor**
**Chemical Bonding     Structure of the Atom**
**Computer     Nuclear Power**

---

***Clocks and clouds.*** At this point it is good to think again in terms of a world that presents itself as a combination of "clocks" and "clouds," the clocks being things and ideas that are definite and well determined, the clouds things and ideas that are vague, fuzzy, and indeterminate. This is our world.

***Chaos theory.*** Chaos theory tells us that in our world we have a state of chaos on the one hand and a state of order on the other. The formation of our universe took place in a state of disorder (chaos and a big bang), and order slowly evolved from this as it expanded. There is an extremely sensitive balance between the two states. Every system in our world is subject to this type of change, ourselves and our minds and bodies included. A chaotic system is one whose final state is extremely sensitive to the initial conditions: if you change the beginning a little, you change the end a lot. The weather and the stockmarket, for example, are chaotic systems that are hard, and not often impossible, to predict!

***Ripples and nudges.*** Minor influences that we call "little ripples" can lead from a state of order to one of disorder. "Little nudges" can lead from disorder back to orderliness. These quite small interferences have an effect out of all proportion to their size. Here are some of the most common ripples and nudges:

| *Ripples:* | *Nudges:* |
|---|---|
| fear | listening and caring |
| anxiety | laughter |
| anger | explaining |
| uncertainty | encouraging |
| boredom | attention |
| hurry | prayer |

***Turbulence.*** This phenomenon has something in common with chaos theory. The shape of an object, a ship or a plane, moving through water or air, can cause the formation of eddies that resist the passage of the object through the medium. Very small structural changes can cause considerable resistance.

---

**Two Additional Factors**
**Chaos theory and turbulence are controlled by**
**little ripples and little nudges.**

---

The nature of these little ripples and little nudges and the ways in which they act will be discussed more fully in subsequent chapters. They are of vital importance in the maintenance of health, both at home and at work, and in the development of a healthy belief system. They function equally in orthodox, alternative, and complementary medicine.

In facing the problems encountered in the fight against ill health and the fight for health, we are continually dealing with an infinite variety of ever-changing combinations of factors. In fact we think in terms of combinations of things rather than in terms of single individual entities. As the Singaporean couturier Frank Benjamin said about his business activities, "It is the combination that is important." This makes our task more difficult but fortunately also a good deal more fascinating and profitable.

We've tried to present the essentials of Newtonian and quantum physics in as simple a form as possible. The reader who wants more information can get it from Paul Davies' book *God and the New Physics*, from John Polkinghorne's *Quarks, Chaos and Christianity*, or from Gary Zukav's *The Dancing Wu Li Masters*. Polkinghorne presents a very balanced view as a scientist, Fellow of the Royal Society, and theologian.

# — 3 —

# The American Back Society

THE FACT THAT I (WHK-W) have been a member of the American Back Society for over ten years and president for three has stimulated me to write about the relationships between orthodox conventional medicine, on the one hand, and many of the branches of complementary and alternative medicine on the other.

This flourishing Society owes its existence to the foresight, faith, and hard work of Aubrey and Nedra Swartz. Their influence has spread widely beyond the membership of the Society and its attendees at the past twenty-five meetings. The Society was inaugurated in 1982 and has since then been imbued with the spirit of cooperation among the disciplines concerned in the management of back pain. Meetings of the society have been held throughout the North American continent, including Buffalo, Cambridge, Chicago, Las Vegas, Los Angeles, Montreal, New Orleans, San Francisco, and Toronto. Attendees at each meeting, numbering several hundred, have come away with the satisfaction of having improved their knowledge and clinical acumen in the field of spinal care. Many health care professionals attending these meetings come from foreign countries as well.

I hope to tell you in subsequent chapters how I became interested in the work of disciplines other than my own of orthodox conventional medicine, first in East Africa and later in North America. Exciting times in these two very different parts of the world have led me to the mountaintop where the spirit of the American Back Society has its rightful place. Great has been my good fortune to be associated closely with the work of this Society.

For some years before 1982 Aubrey and Nedra were disturbed at the inadequate communication among the various disciplines in the back care community. They became aware that there was all too little understanding and tolerance among the disciplines concerned, and that this had an observable adverse effect upon patients suffering from spinal problems, including painful conditions of the neck and back. All too often, the patient was at a disadvantage, due to the confusion and misunderstanding among the various disciplines, and was caught in the crossfire of contemptuous attitudes expressed by those professionals who provided consultation and treatment. To make matters worse, when there was more than one health care provider seeing the patient for the same problem, there was often a lack of effective communication between them. Frequently a health care provider would be at a loss as to whom and to what discipline to refer the patient. Often the provider did not have an adequate understanding of the services provided by the various disciplines concerned with these types of problems. This situation, dismal at it appeared, often took a turn for the worse when the patient was referred to a physician who was not particularly interested in treating back pain.

The goal of the American Back Society was, from the start, to improve understanding, recognition, and respect among the members of the various disciplines concerned and to increase the awareness health care providers had of the training, knowledge, and skills of those in other disciplines. This Society was created as an open scientific forum for all of the various disciplines concerned to come together and learn from one another.

The meetings of the Society have included lectures, panel discussions, question-and-answer sessions from the audience, courses, conferences, workshops, and clinical presentations. ABS Grand Rounds, in which there are clinical case presentations to an expert panel of at least twelve health care professionals representing a wide variety of disciplines in the spinal community, have been one of the highlights of these meetings. The attendees have experienced a rare opportunity to observe how many of these disciplines approach a clinical problem, with respect to diagnosis and treatment. A very interesting observation regarding these case presentations has been that, after an extensive discussion among the panelists, there is frequently a consensus among them with a good measure of agreement as to how these patients should be managed. ABS Grand Rounds, therefore, have demonstrated that an interdisciplinary group, representing a wide range of professions, specialties, and disciplines within the spinal care community, can view these issues in an objective manner and arrive at decisions in the spirit of a cooperative team approach, decisions that also appear to be best for the patient. The message conveyed from all these events is loud and clear. We can work together more effectively as colleagues than as competitors.

The faculty members have always been carefully chosen and have appropriately represented the various disciplines concerned with spinal care. At least half of the attendees have been doctors of medicine and the other half have come from a wide variety of professions, specialties, and disciplines, which include osteopaths, nurses, chiropractors, physical therapists, occupational therapists, exercise physiologists, acupuncturists, and athletic trainers. The Society's meetings have been most worthwhile, and the level of interest and enthusiasm continues to be high among the attendees, faculty, technical exhibitors, and staff at these events.

I have experienced a good deal of gratification from having the opportunity to engage in discussions with many different health care professionals. These discussions might include points of interest or differences, but the exchanges have all been productive, and I have enjoyed the opportunity of becoming good friends with many of the professionals whom I have met at these meetings. I have always looked forward to meeting up once again with these friends and acquaintances at each successive meeting. It has been a truly enjoyable process, learning to appreciate other people's viewpoints, even though different from our own. This aspect of the Society's life and work is to me its true genius.

From these meetings came, for many of us, opportunities to visit spine centers far and wide in North America and occasionally farther afield, sometimes as casual visitors and sometimes as visiting lecturers. In all of these the new idea was spread that the way ahead was through cooperation of physicians and others in many different disciplines in pursuit of their common interest in back pain.

In all the years of being at these meetings, I can only remember one occasion when a physician was unnecessarily unpleasant to someone in another discipline, during the question and answer session. The individual, who was confrontational, was challenged by a senior physician in his own discipline, which then resulted in a good deal of laughter, and things were once again placed in the right perspective. I have enjoyed my professional relationship and friendship with Aubrey, as we have both always felt that the patient with back pain would ultimately benefit from a team approach rather than from any one individual effort.

I've no doubt that Aubrey chose exactly the right moment of time to start the society. A few years earlier would have been too soon, and then the whole project might well have been a failure. As things have turned out, the work of this society has from the start been a great success. It was in the 1980s that interdisciplinary cooperation began to take place and spread all over the North American continent, soon after the inauguration of ABS. At the time of writing one hears nearly every week about some new cooperative project. Universities and medical schools are taking up the challenge. It is perhaps not surprising that the expectations and demands now made by patients and their relatives are some of the main driving forces that encourage those responsible for teaching students, residents, and others seeking to update their skills to promote interdisciplinary cooperation. Symposia on orthodox, complementary, and alternative medicine are now the order of the day. Many of us are very proud of the courage and foresight shown by Aubrey and Nedra Swartz.

We look back several thousand years to the work of the Greek healing centers in Delphi, Epidauros, and Cos, following this by observation of the ways in which the prevention and care of the sick has developed over the centuries to the present time. The picture that presents itself to our eyes is one of steadily progressing cooperation. Time and again physicians and others have been moved by unseen forces to strive to work together. It is as though the Creator foresaw the need for health care before He created the universe and laid down guidelines for us to work together in combination. Indeed this business of putting two or more concerns together to form a combination seems to be part of the warp and woof of the environment in which we live. The work of ABS and other similar ventures is in fact the norm. We are confident that it will continue to blossom and flourish.

# ORTHODOX
# AND
# COMPLEMENTARY
# DISCIPLINES

# — 4 —

# Mainstream Medicine

ONE OF THE EARLIEST kinds of medicine we know was practiced in China from about 3000 B.C. It emphasized the importance of preventive measures and of the oneness of mind and body, things that we are just beginning to relearn today. Hippocrates lived and worked on the Aegean island of Cos about 2500 B.C.. He is now regarded as the father of modern medicine, and his oath is accepted as the modern code of ethics. The Christian monastic movement began about 400 A.D. Before long it embraced the healing art, to a large extent through the use of herbs and herbal potions and salves. The first known medieval medical schools were developed about 1,400 A.D. in Oxford and Cambridge, the Sorbonne in Paris, and the University in Siena. At the British universities it was not long before the first four doctorates in divinity, music, law, and medicine were instituted. Physicians began to have a rightful place in society from that time on.

The Guild of Barber Surgeons followed, two to three hundred years later. Surgical training was at first an apprenticeship inferior to that of physicians, and the surgeon was not entitled to call himself doctor. From this time on physicians and surgeons emphasized bleeding, purging, and cupping, a regime that commended them neither to the authorities in Europe nor to their patients. In the seventeenth and eighteenth centuries a relatively few British physicians in high social circles enjoyed a considerable reputation, though their rural counterparts were not highly regarded.

The advance of medicine on the North American continent lagged behind that in Europe. The German physician Hahnemann introduced homeopathy about 1790 A.D. as an antidote to the crude practices of the orthodox physicians of the time. In North America homeopathy was accepted quite quickly, and homeopathic hospitals and medical schools were built. In 1875 there were thousands of homeopathic physicians and millions of adherents. In its heyday homeopathy was a serious alternative to the regular schools. It enjoyed a high reputation, mainly due to the effective way in which it treated serious infectious diseases such as typhoid fever. The results obtained by this new discipline were much better than those of the conventional medicine of the day.

In 1864 the American physician Andrew Taylor Still rejected orthodox medicine when he lost three children to a meningitis epidemic despite heroic treatment. He developed great interest in alternative methods of healing and invented osteopathy, which went a considerable way to counter the ineffective attempts of the M.D. physician to deal with rheumatic and rheumatoid conditions. It was late toward the end of the nineteenth century that Simpson discovered chloroform as an anesthetic, Semmelweiss discovered the way to control puerperal sepsis, Pasteur discovered the role of bacteria in postoperative infections, and Lister discovered how to perform antiseptic surgery, using a carbolic acid spray, which kept the operative site germ-free. (It incidentally made the urine passed by the surgeon and his assistants green in color, much to their initial alarm.)

The discovery of anesthetics and the introduction of first antiseptic and later aseptic surgery heralded great advancement in the practice of surgery. Previous to these discoveries surgery was greatly feared by the patient, and with reason, for it was extremely painful, and serious infection was often lethal. Lister was the first, initially in Glasgow and later in London, to make operative surgery relatively safe and reliable. Today we would regard the surgery of those days as being very primitive.

Toward the end of the eighteenth and for the first part of the nineteenth century the standing of the medical profession was, on the whole, not high. Conventional medicine underwent a difficult period of transition in the second half of the nineteenth century. It was regarded as being very primitive. Before the Civil War there was considerable distrust of the regular medical schools. A Popular Health Movement, led largely by women, poured scorn on the way in which physicians and surgeons went about their work. At this time there were two alternative movements. The first, under Samuel Thomson, was a reconstructed system of folk medicine that claimed four million adherents. The second, under Sylvester Graham, advocated a diet of raw fruit and vegetables and whole grains. The only remaining vestige of this movement is the graham cracker.

Conditions for doctors in North America lagged behind those in Europe. The discovery in the last century by the veterinary surgeon Jenner that purulent material from cows with cowpox—when injected into the human skin, protected the patient from the lethal scourge smallpox—introduced the era of immunization, which continues to blossom and is such an important part of preventive medicine today. One of the most important discoveries in medicine and it was made by a veterinary surgeon! This discovery by someone who was not a medical man did much to boost the standing of the medical profession. It is fascinating to think that the practice of surgery owes as much to the nonsurgeons Semellweiss, Pasteur, and Simpson as to surgeons like Lister and the Mayo brothers.

At the beginning of the eighteenth century attempts were made, first in Europe and rather later in North America, to register medical practitioners. Over the next hundred years emphasis on controlling practitioners by registration waxed and waned. Homeopathic hospitals in the U.S. 152 years ago had by far the best record for treating infections such as typhoid fever. From the middle of the nineteenth century onward, requirements for registration were more strictly controlled. At this time, in 1846, members of the conventional medical profession organized themselves to form the American Medical Association. They quickly came to regard themselves as the premier discipline and excluded practitioners in other kinds of disciplines. They were unwilling to accept midwives. They discouraged their members from developing contacts with homeopathic physicians, a move that made caused difficulties for the latter, threatening the continuing existence of homeopathic hospitals.

The attitude of the AMA to osteopathic physicians was at first inimical, but early in the twentieth century the two professions, conventional and osteopathic medicine, resolved their differences and formed an alliance. The result was that the M.D. and the D.O. degrees became interchangeable. In the process many osteopaths ceased to practice as such, conforming completely to conventional therapy and ceasing to practice osteopathy. In North America and in Great Britain there are still a number of groups of qualified osteopaths who continue to practice osteopathic medicine of very high caliber, often in cooperation with practitioners of mainstream medicine.

Relations between the chiropractic profession and the American Medical Association had not been satisfactory for a number of years. Litigation ensued in the mid-nineteenth century between the AMA and the chiropractic profession. Finally in 1987 a U.S. District Court judge ruled that the AMA and its officials were guilty of attempting to eliminate the Chiropractic profession. This ruling was confirmed by the U.S. Supreme Court in 1990. In 1991 the AMA agreed to make a considerable contribution toward the chiropractic legal costs and to revise its position. One result of this was that mainstream medicine began to acknowledge that there might be something of value in chiropractic and in other forms of complementary medicine. A similar dispute between the American Nurses Association and the AMA is not yet completely resolved. American medical societies are still critical of all disciplines that are outside the purview of conventional medicine. There is a continual shift toward increasing cooperation between the various disciplines.

In North America the Mayo brothers did much to foster the initial high standing of the practice of surgery. Their father emigrated from Great Britain toward the end of the nineteenth century, and on arrival in the U.S. moved west to set up general practice in Rochester, Minnesota. He became interested in surgery at a time when this specialty was about to take great leaps forward. He operated on the kitchen table in his home with considerable success. His two sons both qualified as doctors and soon developed their father's interests.

The story is told of how the sons stole their father's thunder. The father left town to attend a medical meeting elsewhere. After the meeting he brought home to Rochester a friend who wanted to see him perform an operation for the removal of an ovarian cyst. He discovered that his two sons had already done this operation themselves. The friend was much more impressed and amused than the father! The three of them, father and sons, proceeded to lay the foundation of the world-renowned Mayo Clinic.

From then on surgery became more respectable and highly regarded on both sides of the Atlantic. In Britain the new king, Edward VI, gave impetus to the development of surgery by developing a case of acute appendicitis just before his coronation. The coronation was postponed. Sir Frederick Treves operated on the king in his bed in the palace. The operation was successful and the king's recovery uneventful. The diagnosis of acute appendicitis became a popular one, and many an aspiring surgeon, as we shall see later, had good reason to thank Sir Frederick. The great man himself was rewarded by a knighthood, given a free house in the Royal Park for life, and gained his main distinction by encouraging Sir Wilfred Grenfell to start his mission in Labrador.

It was not all plain sailing. Early attempts were often crude and the results uncertain. In New York the well-known American surgeon Halstead devised a disfiguring and brutal operation for cancer of the breast which we now know to be ineffective in most cases. In Britain Arbuthnot Lane pioneered the treatment of fractures by open reduction and internal fixation with steel plates and screws, using a nontouch technique to reduce the chance of infection. Unfortunately later in life Sir Arbuthnot became obsessed by an idea, a figment of his imagination, that many cases of general ill health were due to absorption of toxic substances from the colon. For the treatment of this condition he embarked on the mutilating operation of total removal of the colon. Eventually his name was struck off the register of practicing physicians.

But there has been progress. Now the prospective surgeon undergoes many years of postgraduate training in general and special surgery. These are tough years, during which the candidate is at the beck and call of surgeons day and night, often with no time for recreation or for family life. As a result there is an inevitable tendency for the surgeon to think when training is finished, "which one of all the operations with which I am familiar can I perform on this patient?" In cardiology the surgeon is restrained by a physician, the cardiologist. Cardiologists and cardiac surgeons sit down together to discuss the pros and cons of operative intervention. It would be good if there were similar professional groupings appointed to act as safeguards in other fields.

Among some of the most effective drugs that were available came from nature: digitalis, to control the heart rate, from the foxglove; salicylic acid (aspirin), to control pain and fever, from the bark of the willow tree; and quinine from cinchona bark to treat malaria. Had it not been for the open-mindedness of the medical profession, digitalis would have remained a folk remedy outside of conventional medicine. Up to the 1930s the majority of prescriptions, usually dispensed by the physician, consisted of three or four different components, measured in minims and drachms. It was difficult to understand the rationale for substances like syrup of squills or syrup of tolu or tincture of cardamoms! In the 1930s I (WHK-W) and my costudents had to learn to prescribe these and other similar drugs if we wished to obtain the qualification required to practice medicine. We had no idea that much of what we had to learn was nonsense.

Fortunately at this time Bayer in Germany and May and Baker in England produced the first sulphonamides with strong antibacterial properties—Prontosil and M and B 125 and 693. These revolutionized the practice of medicine. By administrating these synthetic drugs, the death rate from lobar pneumonia and from puerperal sepsis was greatly reduced. It is amusing to recall that initially physicians were suspicious of these drugs, thinking that they obscured the symptoms, while all the time they were curing the patient. The discovery of penicillin by Fleming and Florey heralded a new era. Streptomycin and other antibacterial fungal chemicals followed shortly. The factories in which these substances were fermented looked just like breweries, with their large fermenting bins. New pharmaceutical companies appeared like mushrooms to synthesize products in the laboratory which now have such a potent effect on many disease processes. New substances were produced and tested by a process of combinatorial chemistry.

The use of naturally occurring plant products has been largely replaced in recent years by the synthetic drugs produced by pharmaceutical companies. There is now a strong movement to return to the use of naturally occurring products in combination with valuable synthetic drugs. Health stores are common in every town, small or large. Traditional pharmacies now commonly stock their shelves with vitamins and herbal preparations. Practitioners in orthodox medicine now recognize that there is a strong populist movement of empowered consumers toward natural medicine and new techniques.

## Medical Schools and Their Students

It is perhaps not out of place to digress a little to mention something of the conditions under which medical students worked in the United States. At the turn of the century both the public and academia were sceptical of the standards of allopathic medicine throughout the country. The dean and teaching staff at Harvard University Medical School were moved to do what they could to raise the standards in its alliance of colleges. Previous to this, the final qualifying exams were not much more than five-minute orals. They were replaced, with some difficulty, by written exams, though the teaching staff greatly doubted the ability of many students to write intelligible English.

A layman, Abraham Flexner, supported by the Rockefellers, made an indictment of medical education throughout the country in about 1910, which eventually led to the emergence of regular medical schools of a reasonable standard, with a rather rigid, set syllabus that even so was a considerable improvement. With the help of the AMA Flexner pressed for an increase in the standards of premedical education in the sciences. The teaching was often unscientific and in the main determined by the patriarchal system that dictated them.

In the United Kingdom in the 1930s the staff, physicians, and surgeons who gave their services free were like gods, worshiped by the priestesses (the nursing sisters in charge of wards), supported by the residents, and sustained by the slave labor of the students, an unnecessary evil that not even the Greek gods on Mount Parnasus would have perpetrated. The following incident speaks for itself. The surgeon in cap, gown, and gloves, fierce with bushy eyebrows and piercing eyes peering over the mask that covered most of his face, dropped his scalpel on the theater floor and fixed the new student with his penetrating gaze. Looking back and forth from student to scalpel, he suggested silently that the wretched student, also in sterile cap, gown, and gloves, pick up the scalpel from the nonsterile floor. Eventually the unfortunate young man bent down and picked up the scalpel. At this all hell broke loose, as the surgeon yelled at him, cursing him that in sterile clothing he dared to contaminate himself by touching a nonsterile object, and shouting at him in the most abusive terms to get out and stay out of his theater. The wretched student was a fellow student of mine. I might well have been that student!

There were surgeons who were less unkind, but few if any of them took the trouble to teach the slave labor much, if anything. Students were there to hold retractors for the surgeon or to write notes about the operation for him. On one occasion the surgeon, dictating the findings as he opened the abdominal cavity in a male patient said, "Right ovary normal, left ovary normal . . ." This was known as retractology! It consumed hours of the students' time for two three-month periods.

Teaching on the surgical wards was equally unhelpful. We learned to take it with resignation. I remember saying to myself, "I can't do anything about this now, but if ever I'm in general practice near London, I'll never, ever refer a patient to these surgeons." One of us, a commander invalided out of the Navy, older and tougher than the rest of us, went to complain to the dean, who received him graciously and promised to deal with our complaint, but we never experienced any signs of change of surgical heart. This attitude on the part of our teachers is surprising, given medicine's frequent claims of the unsatisfactory and unscientific nature of the teaching given in the schools of complementary and alternative medicine. Orthodox medicine was and perhaps often still is in the same or even a more leaking boat.

Fortunately there was another side to the coin, which was as bright as the first was dull and depressing. I was introduced to a brilliant surgeon at another hospital who took the trouble to teach me a great deal. As his clinical load grew greater, Robert McNeill Love had insufficient time to run his Boy Scout district in the London dock area. As a medical student I became his assistant in scouting. In exchange he taught me the principles of surgery, and he was the person who inspired me to become a surgeon. He was the best teacher I have ever met. The other surgeons at the teaching hospital barred his election to the staff. It was thought by many that this was because he was more able than they were and would attract their patients, to their financial detriment! He and a friend, Hamilton Bailey, produced a short textbook of surgery that was much better than similar long books from other surgeons. It was very popular but disliked by other surgeons, who referred to it in a derogatory way as "the little book"!

When criticizing the surgeon today, it is necessary to remember the appalling state of the practice of this art two centuries ago, before the advent of anesthesia and antiseptic surgery. The tasks demanded so much of those who practiced them that great toughness was required. One of these was the French surgeon Duputyren, who was renowned for his disregard for human suffering. A poor Parisian woman, about to have an amputation of the leg without any anesthetic, was shaking with fear. Dupytren came up to her and said, "What are you worried about? Don't you realize that the great Dupytren is going to operate on you?"

The physicians, more gentle and kindly individuals, did make some effort to teach us, but they were quite unpredictable. In my first week on a medical ward the physician asked to see my notes on a patient, perused them briefly, and grunted, "Young man you'll never make a doctor, your writing is too good. You should try journalism." It was easy to correct that deficiency! During the next week one physician told us that a low-protein diet was mandatory in a case of chronic nephritis. The next day another physician said that for this condition a high-protein diet was essential. Did they not know or did they not care? It probably didn't matter anyway. One of these young men later became physician to the king and queen, but as far as I know they never suffered from nephritis! One or two of the physicians were brilliant teachers. At their teaching rounds on the wards so many students crowded round the patient's bed that it was difficult to see or hear anything. Pity the poor patient who got free treatment from the cream of the medical crop. It was difficult for him or her to feel like a human being.

Teaching on pathology and on microbiology was very good. That on psychiatry was good but depressing. That about preventive medicine was conspicuous by its absence. We never heard a word about medical ethics. I ask myself what, if anything, we learned from those three years in the hospital. I think the chief things were those we absorbed without realizing it by a process of osmosis. One couldn't have acquired an inkling about what it means to be a doctor in any other way than by submitting, albeit unwillingly, to the frustrations and humiliations of life in a teaching hospital in the 1930s. If we complained that something was unfair, we were told, "This is good preparation for you, because life in general is unfair"! I wonder if it's any better now?

The actual knowledge required to enable us to pass the written examinations was gained by the individual's reading. This depended on one's ability to make good, careful notes of lectures and of what one read in the evening back in one's digs. By no means all of us had this ability. We were taught the mechanics of how to talk to the patient and how to examine him or her. These things were demonstrated to us by our teachers. Few of these taught us that a patient is a human being. To them a patient was an object to which a disease entity was attached. These things we had to learn for ourselves, and some of us took a long time to do so. There was little if any attention given to the effect of the home or the workplace on the sick person.

Without saying anything, our teachers gave us a very clear message—that there was no way of treating a sick person other than by the kind of medicine we were learning. There were unfortunately a few cranks about the place, but we needn't pay any attention to them.

The second unspoken message, one that was very definite, was that when we became doctors we would have the world at our feet. It would be the very ungrateful patient who didn't appreciate our efforts. If someone died, it wasn't our responsibility. The result of this attitude was that doctors didn't like to have contact with patients who were dying or with their relatives. This task was left to the head nurse, the ward sister. There were exceptions. The senior neurologist was a man who seemed to be aloof from students, always in a hurry, belching a good deal during his lectures and apparently much concerned with making the last buck. We discovered by accident that he came back to the hospital every Sunday afternoon to chat with patients and their relatives, moving from bed to bed, apparently in no hurry at all.

The final examinations for students from Cambridge were held back in that city. The pass rate was about fifty percent. This exam was a real hurdle. It was held twice a year. One could go back to take it as often as one liked! I counted myself fortunate to scrape through at the first attempt. For general practice in the 1930s no internship was required. Fortunately that omission has long since been remedied. Malpractice insurance with and membership of the General Medical Council was the princely sum of ten pounds sterling a year.

## The Past Fifty Years

In the early years of this century the emphasis was much more on hygiene and prevention. More was accomplished by mainstream and conventional medicine in improving the water supply and dealing with sewage and sanitation than in any other field. The role of immunization increased considerably to include preventive measures against smallpox, diphtheria, typhoid, and poliomyelitis. These and other similar measures have done so much to improve the health of people all over the world. Physicians concerned with these matters deserve the highest praise. It is likely that they have done more to improve the health of the people in Britain, Europe, the United States, and elsewhere than anyone else.

The days in 1934 and 1935 when the first antibiotics appeared on the market were most exciting. The initial discovery was made by the German company Bayer, maker of aniline dyes, who found that adding a sulphur radical to the dye gave it antibacterial properties. The result was Prontosil. In England the pharmaceutical firm May and Baker soon after this produced other antibacterial drugs, M and B 125 and M and B 693. These discoveries were revolutionary. Many serious infections responded to these drugs, including pneumococcal pneumonia, puerperal sepsis, meningitis, and postoperative infections. It is impossible to overestimate the excitement produced by the availability of these drugs.

During two weeks on the hospital wards in 1938 I (WHK-W) heard an obstetrician say, "This woman with a severe postpartum infection is going to live, she's on Prontosil." And a surgeon on the infectious disease ward, "This patient has a lethal anthrax infection, a boil at the back of the neck, caught from cattle on the farm. He's on M and B 693, and I think he'll live." And a physician on a medical ward, "This man with lobar pneumonia is on the new drug M and B 125. His temperature came down from 103 degrees to normal this morning and he looks well, but I'm worried that the drug has masked the symptoms." (It hadn't.) These were indeed stirring days for conventional medicine. It took us a while to appreciate the terrific advance.

Over the next few years several other sulphonamides came on the market. The early 1940s saw the release of penicillin, made from the fungus that grows on jams, discovered by Fleming and Florey. At first this new wonder drug was available only to the armed forces during the second World War, but before long it was available for civilians too. It was not long before streptomycin was discovered, to reduce greatly the menace of tuberculous infections. Many other antibiotics soon followed.

Not until thirty years later did our profession begin to realize that, due mainly to the indiscriminate use of antibiotics, many pathogenic organisms which were initially sensitive to antibiotics had developed resistance. The problem of resistant strains has been particularly bad in hospitals. Many patients now develop infections in the hospital who had none before admission. A number of these infections are resistant to many antibiotics. The problem is very severe in cases of tuberculosis. We thought we had got the better of this infection, but today this is far from the truth.

The most serious infection at present is a necrotizing fasciitis and myositis due to a virulent strain of streptococcus. It is not uncommon for patients with this condition to lose life or limb. We call to mind the mythical story of Hercules and the Hydra. Every time the warrior cut off one head, three new heads took its place. Eventually as Hercules cut off a head he cauterized the stump with a brand from the fire. In this way he finally killed the dragon. To deal with resistant infections today calls for equal persistence and ingenuity. An article in one of the American journals in 1994 stated that over two million patients in hospital developed drug reactions while there, and over 100,000 died as a result.

For brevity, we do no more than mention other striking advances: complex physical and operative techniques for the treatment of fractures and other severe injuries; the effective management of emergencies; the elaboration of new and often complicated surgical techniques, including brain, heart, chest, reconstructive joint, and particularly replacement has made tremendous strides. The treatment of diabetes was taught us by an enthusiastic but rather uninspiring elderly physician, who had taken the trouble to study under Banting and Best in Toronto. Preventive medicine and surgery were given much more attention; prospective double blind trials were instituted; an attempt was made to assess comparative costs of treatment. It must be admitted that the great majority of medical and surgical treatments have not yet been assessed for the effect of treatment and for cost-effectiveness.

What are the things that mainstream, conventional medicine does well?

1. Immunization through the development of vaccines
2. Use of antibiotics to control infections
3. Treatment of trauma, reconstructive surgery, and joint replacement
4. Management of emergencies
5. Control and treatment of diabetes
6. Anesthesia and asepsis
7. Surgical techniques for brain surgery, open-heart surgery, and other operations
8. Diagnostic techniques
9. Double-blind controlled trials
10. Promotion of scientific biomedical research

What are the areas in which conventional medicine needs improvement?

1. Preventive medicine, apart from immunization
2. Treatment of cancer
3. Treatment of common musculoskeletal problems
4. Rapport with the patient
5. Treating the patient as a whole person
6. Practice of evidence-based health care

# A New Era

We are now spectators at the birth of a new era, due largely to dissatisfaction expressed by the public with several aspects of orthodox medicine. Patients are no longer prepared to wait to see the specialist, nor for admission to hospital. No longer do they take every word of the physician as gospel truth: they want a say in the decision as to the best treatment. They demand the right to seek alternative treatment. As a result medical practitioners are now more willing to cooperate with those in complementary medicine, reluctant though some may still be. This heralds the dawn of a new era of cooperation between the disciplines of mainstream medicine and complementary alternatives, which will almost certainly result in a form of treatment that is more cost-effective, more

efficient, more pleasant for the patient, and more enjoyable for all the physicians concerned.

When orthodox physicians and surgeons gained full recognition during the last century, a strong tendency developed over the ensuing years for them to become arrogant and overbearing. This is now in the process of being corrected. There is a similar danger that practitioners in the newly liberated disciplines of complementary and alternative medicine will, in their turn, become overconfident, arrogant, and overbearing. To be aware of this possibility is to check the tendency in its infancy, something of extreme importance for all of us. All too often success breeds arrogance and intolerance.

Let's look at what do those in complementary medicine do better.

1. They have shown more interest in promoting health and preventing disease. They aim at a healthy lifestyle.
2. They are convinced of the value of treating the whole person.
3. They are aware that there are two phases in the recovery of a sick person—the treatment necessary to cure or alleviate the disease process and helping the patient to feel better.
4. They support the treatment of cancer and other terminal illnesses, using techniques such as guided imagery.
5. They are less involved in complex diagnostic and therapeutic techniques and so have more time to give the patient personal attention.
6. They treat some musculoskeletal conditions more effectively.
7. Sometimes they are more cost-effective.

Where do those in complementary medicine need to improve?

1. Sometimes they offer false hope to those with incurable diseases.
2. On occasion they hide behind vitalistic theories, almost relinquishing the responsibility of carrying out research to validate the efficacy of their treatment.
3. Some tend to oversimplify the pathophysiological basis of disease and overstate the potential benefits of their therapies.

In the prevention and treatment of disease processes there is room for many different disciplines and no impelling reason to fear competition from others. There is a need for all physicians and therapists to learn about the way that others work, whether it be in mainstream or in complementary fields. This need can be met in two ways: by including teaching about the work of other disciplines in the curriculum of the discipline concerned, and by seminars and conferences designed for people of many different disciplines. The American Back Society, with its annual meetings for all comers, has over the past ten years done a splendid job in this respect.

Some examples of schools that teach about alternative medicine are: Harvard Medical School; University of British Columbia, Alternative Medicines in Pharmacy Practice; Tzu Chi Institute in Vancouver; Stanford University, Complementary and Alternative Medicine; University of Minnesota Medical School, Addiction and Alternative Medicine Research; University of California at Davis, Alternative Medicine Research in Asthma and Immunology; University of Texas Health Science Center, Alternative Medicine and Cancer Research; Palmer College, Davenport, Iowa, Consortial Center for Chiropractic Research; University of Virginia, Study of Complementary and Alternative Therapies; University of Maryland School of Medicine, Alternative Medicine Pain Research and Evaluation; Bastyr University AIDS Research Center in Washington; Columbia University, Alternative and Complementary Medicine Research.

# My Medical Practice

For the whole of my (WHK-W) time in medical school and for the first seven years of medical practice in East Africa, I was fully occupied in learning and then putting into practice my knowledge of orthodox, mainstream medicine and surgery. After the first year in East Africa, at a place called Kaloleni, near Mombasa, I was responsible for the medical and surgical work of a hospital of fifty beds, including obstetrics. This was a tough experience, which included dealing with a young man who'd been gored by a rhinoceros whose horn penetrated both rectum and bladder; inserting a bone graft to treat an older man who'd been attacked by a buffalo and who managed to escape by climbing a tree with a broken clavicle; operating on a woman who said she'd been pregnant for seven years but could not deliver her baby—she had in fact an immense ovarian cyst the size of a nine month pregnancy!

More difficult was the problem of how to deal with a woman on whom a witch doctor had cast a death spell. We gave her a very large dose of paraldehyde to put her to sleep for eight hours, and when she woke up an immense dose of Epsom salts, which sent her frequently to the toilet to evacuate the evil spirits. She survived, and her husband was surprised and delighted. Was this an ethical way of managing the case? One can look back and laugh now, but it was not so funny for a young, inexperienced surgeon at the time. The last two examples tell us that it is essential to take into account anthropological and sociological factors that are strange to the Western mind. Success here depended on some understanding of the way the African person thought about herself and her environment.

After the first five years in East Africa, my days were fully occupied by routine orthopedics in a hospital with a hundred orthopedic beds, helped by one resident and one intern. This full-time job was combined with prescribing and supervising manipulation of the low back, helped first by one and later by several physical therapists. This proved to be a heavy workload but an excellent introduction to a future practice that combined routine orthodox medicine and surgery with alternative and complementary medicine. Little did I think that the things I learned in Africa under primitive conditions would be such good training for the integration of orthodox and complementary medicine in a North American environment. My interest in the spine was kindled by the fact that I spent so much time in Africa treating bone and joint tuberculosis, of which the spine was an important part. In Saskatchewan infections of the spine were uncommon, so I looked around for a new interest and became quickly engrossed in the management of neck and low-back pain. Hence the absorbing interest in the cooperation of many different disciplines.

# – 5 –

# Homeopathy

IN PHARMACIES THAT SELL natural health products in North America, the customer sees row upon row of homeopathic medicines, often with a note indicating their uses. There they are amongst many rows of more conventional over-the-counter drugs, vitamins, and other health products. If the shopper pauses to look around, he or she will spot other customers browsing and inspecting one product after another and taking two or three bottles to the counter to pay for them. Many people today apparently get a lot of satisfaction, rightly or wrongly, from deciding what medications they need for their health. Vitamins and minerals seem to be much in demand.

French pharmacies must stock and sell homeopathic medicines by law. We're told that they sell faster than they can be replaced. About thirty percent of family practitioners in France prescribe homeopathic drugs, and rather more than thirty percent use them. There are medical schools in France that give postgraduate degrees in homeopathy.

The name homeopathy comes from two Greek words, *homoios*, similar, and *pathos*, suffering. Nearly all kinds of healing have their origin in Chinese, Indian, or Greek medicine. And so it was with homeopathy, which was first practiced by a German physician, Samuel Hahnemann, about 1790. Hahnemann got his ideas from Hippocrates, who noticed in the fourth century B.C. that large quantities of certain natural herbs and other similar products could produce symptoms that resembled those caused by disease. He also noticed that small doses of the same substance could relieve the symptoms, and that very small amounts of substances obtained from plants could enhance the body's resistance to some disease processes.

Hahnemann took these findings and worked them up into his own concept—homeopathy. He made the observation that tiny amounts of some plant and animal substances sometimes led to an increased resistance to illness. He experimented on himself, taking quinine from the chincona bark, and produced the symptoms of malaria. This he treated to his satisfaction by taking small doses of quinine. His theory was that small doses of herbs and other substances stimulated the defense mechanisms of the body. Hippocrates had postulated that if a substance caused disease, then a like substance would bring a cure. Hahnemann called this the *law of similars*. The well-known Swiss physician Paracelsus had much the same idea, expressed rather differently.

Later on Hahnemann formulated another law, of *infinitesimals*: the more dilute the substance the stronger its healing power. The process of dilution was termed *succussion*. The fluid was diluted to such an extent that it had virtually nothing left of the original substance. He also firmly believed that the body has a "life force," but this has never been demonstrated scientifically.

Hahnemann was stimulated to formulate his theory and put it into practice, because he was so disgusted by the brutal treatment advocated by the so-called conventional system of treatment of disease of the day—cupping, bleeding, purging, and other similarly crude methods.

Homeopathy had a successful launching and rapidly spread throughout Europe and across the Atlantic to the United States. Curiously enough, members of the Royal Family in Britain were impressed, and they have been treated for several generations by physicians who practice homeopathic medicine.

On its introduction to the United States at the end of the eighteenth century homeopathy gained an excellent reputation due to its success in treating many of the epidemics of that century such as cholera, scarlet fever and typhoid. The mortality rates from those infections in homeopathic hospitals were less than half of the rates in conventional hospitals.

Homeopathic physicians had their own approach to sickness and disease. Amongst other things they thought that orthodox medicine relied too much on drugs, which in their opinion often masked the symptoms and caused more serious problems.

Homeopathy prospered in the United States, as it had in Europe, for more than half of the nineteenth century. The discipline attracted wealthy patrons who were prepared to endow a number of homeopathic hospitals. In this way homeopathy was able to attain respectability within the body of the medical profession, even though its physicians held what many would call unorthodox opinions.

At the founding of the American Medical Association in the middle years of the nineteenth century, a clause in the code of ethics discouraged its members from seeking consultation with homeopaths. From then on life was tough for members of the profession. When President Abraham Lincoln was shot and Seward, the Secretary of State was stabbed, the U.S. Surgeon General rushed to help them, but he was strongly denounced for consulting with a homeopath, Seward's physician. The A.M.A. fought homeopaths, not on a matter of principle, as far as we can tell, but to get their business and put money in the bank—a battle waged for purely financial reasons.

After the Flexner report in 1910 (a report made by a civil servant who was not medically qualified) most of these hospitals were forced to close their doors. Many homeopathic hospitals were compelled to accept the teaching and practice of conventional orthodox medicine. The Hahnemann Hospital in Philadelphia, bearing the name of the founder, is the only remaining one in North America.

Still later, not long ago in the twentieth century, national and international bodies belatedly recognized, or at the very least sanctioned, the practice of homeopathy. People in Europe and in American spend billions of euros and dollars each year on homeopathic medicines.

**Definitions.** Right from the beginning of time every system of medicine has had a mental, spiritual, virtual aspect on the one hand and a down-to-earth physical aspect on the other. This is to be expected, because human beings are made up of a combination of these two, the mental and the physical. Unconsciously we think in terms of the mental-physical combo in every aspect and situation of our lives. Hahnemann thought of the mental aspect in terms of what he called the "life force," though we very much doubt whether he could come down to earth to explain it clearly and definitely. The physical aspect of his proposition was represented by the process of succussion on which he laid so much emphasis, once again without much scientific backing.

**Criticism and Defense.** There has been much criticism of Hahnemann's postulates, because the dilution of the agents, as recommended by him, was so great that the original substance was almost nonexistent and this inert pharmacologically. The larger the number of digits before the name of the product, the greater the dilution. Hahnemann thought that these original substances were still active biologically and able to stimulate the immune system. These ideas of his later gained support from the work of the veterinary surgeon William Jenner, who immunized patients against smallpox by administering intradermally a very small dose of purulent material from a case of cowpox, a disease of cattle similar to smallpox but quite benign in men and women. Jenner thought that the antigens of smallpox and cowpox were similar, and that the cowpox antigen was able to produce sufficient antibody to kill the very harmful virus.

In retrospect it is best to regard Hahnemann's work as a reaction to a system that preceded it. It was an escape to a new and better world and at the time a very successful one.

**The Pharmacopoeia.** The first list of substances was drawn up about 1897. It was composed of herbs and similar substances such as dried flowers, roots of plants, berries, seeds, and foods like honey. In 1938 the United

States Congress passed a law legitimizing the use of homeopathic drugs. This was done very much against the wishes and advice and considerably to the annoyance of the orthodox medical community, which must have felt that homeopathy had the edge on conventional medicine and resented this.

There are now a large number of homeopathic remedies, mostly obtained from flowers and plants. In favor of homeopathy is the fact that very small amounts of agents that cause allergic reactions, when injected intradermally, can prevent future occurrence of those reactions. Recently it has been found that a small dose of aspirin is more effective than a large one in preventing clotting of the blood in the blood vessels.

**Diagnosis.** For the homeopathic physician the process of diagnosis has always been complex, involving an assessment of the patient's lifestyle, taking into account the patent's environment, state of mind, personality, and family history. This is a very time-consuming process. Recently use has been made of the computer in making this very thorough assessment. In fact in this respect homeopathy has been ahead of orthodox medicine, whose practitioners are now belatedly becoming aware of the importance of the patient's psychological makeup and of his or her surroundings.

**Treatment.** Homeopathic practitioners are often also M.D.s who, after qualifying, give more attention than usual to lifestyle, the environment, and the patient's personality than the ordinary M.D. does. They do not seem to encounter any great difficulty in a combined approach. Some French medical schools offer a postgraduate qualification in homeopathy.

Homeopathic practitioners usually give only one medication for a particular set of symptoms, but may sometimes give a combination of substances. They believe most of us are overmedicated and that we need to be "detoxified," stressing the point that toxic reactions to orthodox medicines are responsible for one third of all admissions to hospital each year. These dicta appear reasonable enough. (What the homeopath disliked strongly were the methods used for detoxification by orthodox medicine—cupping, bleeding, and purging.)

It is when homeopaths claim to be able to cure almost any disorder from asthma to back pain that people like ourselves become suspicious of

---

their work. The homeopathic physician's claim that the body possesses a vital force that responds to minute doses of natural substances presents a similar problem for orthodox investigators, who have never been able to demonstrate the existence of that force.

We have to admit that in a serious acute emergency, such as myocardial infarction or acute appendicitis, the patient should be referred immediately to an orthodox physician or surgeon who is skilled in dealing with it. We cannot go along with the claim that nearly every disorder can be dealt with by the administration of homeopathic remedies, but we do approve of the fact that there are few side effects to these medications.

***Scientific Evidence.*** Much support for the effectiveness of homeopathic treatment is anecdotal. Reviewers of more than one hundred studies done by homeopathic physicians thought that these did not meet scientific standards. One study on the treatment of asthma published in *The Lancet* some years ago appeared to demonstrate that homeopathic treatment was more effective than that obtained by a placebo. A double-blind study in the same journal on the management of hay fever showed that with homeopathic substances less antihistamine was required than with a placebo. In these studies homeopathic drugs were compared to placebos rather than to other conventional drugs.

***Acceptance of Homeopathy.*** Many orthodox practitioners in the United States consider that homeopathy is no more than an exercise in the use of placebos, but we have to admit that the effects of the latter are often powerful. It is a curious fact that, in spite of this, the orthodox physician tolerates the homeopathic community for all but life-threatening conditions, though he does not routinely refer patients to homeopaths. The World Health Organization recognizes homeopathy as an effective type of conventional medicine, and many other national bodies throughout the world sanction its use. Citizens of North American countries spend billions of dollars each year on homeopathic medicines at health stores as well as at regular pharmacies.

An M.D. homeopath would most likely say that we should let the patient make the decision as to which kind of physician he or she wishes to go for help. Orthodox practitioners are perhaps rather inclined to be intolerant of others and annoyed when the patient wishes to seek help form homeopaths and others. It is perhaps more important that the patient choose to whom he goes for treatment than anything else. This brings us back to the quantum finding that the observer and the observed are closely connected, the former markedly influencing the latter. In view of this, the best advice one can give any patient is, "If you don't feel happy and at ease with your doctor, conventional, homeopathic, or other, change and get help from someone else." It still holds good that we should advise the patient to go to the appropriate well-trained specialist for the treatment of serious accidents, emergencies, and life-threatening conditions.

In an earlier chapter when thinking about quantum mechanics, chaos theory, and the effects of turbulence, we realized that very small initial changes in any system can lead to very big changes at the end. Very small deleterious changes, little ripples, could lead to chaos, and equally small beneficial influences, little nudges, could reverse the process. Perhaps we could say that the very dilute natural substances of homeopathy are in a sense like little nudges? This sort of approach strikes us as being the best possible defense so far produced for homeopathy. We have learned that the causes of disease are sometimes Newtonian and sometimes quantum in nature. We can, for example, talk about clocks and clouds. Frequently a clinical situation presents both clocks and clouds in combination. An M.D. physician who is also a homeopath might well say, "In my work I have sometimes to think as an orthodox physician, sometimes as homeopath, and more often as both in combination." We're right back again to quantum!

***A Tentative Conclusion.*** Homeopathy has made a comeback. Members of the public are for the most part willing to accept this discipline as a reasonable one and prospective patients are prepared to consider going to a homeopath for treatment. Many paying agencies the world over are prepared to deal with homeopaths. The World Health Organization fully recognizes this discipline. Numerous medical and surgical organizations seem content to go along with homeopathy without making a fuss, even if they do not fully endorse its tenets.

# — 6 —

# Chiropractic

M Y (WHK-W) INTRODUCTION first to spinal manipulation and later to chiropractic came out of the blue at the hands of a physician trained in the United Kingdom in conventional medicine and in the United States in osteopathy. He came from London in the mid 1940s to Nairobi to practise manipulative therapy there in private practice. He was introduced to me by a mutual friend, an orthopedic surgeon in London, and he kindly offered to give me and a physical therapist who worked with me some instruction in manipulation of the lumbar spine. This was in fact my introduction to osteopathy, which later led to detailed exposure to chiropractic medicine in Canada.

In the mid-1940s I left the Anglican Mission Hospital near Mombasa, where I'd been working for the past three years, and got a job with the Kenya Medical Department at the Central Hospital in Nairobi. The work in the mission hospital had been very good for me. It had been a tough job, but I'd learned a lot, particularly how to make do with the simplest equipment. Then I felt it was time to move on. My briefing from my new boss, the senior surgical specialist, was to treat all fractures and other injuries in male patients and to run a rehabilitation center for Africans discharged from the army with some continuing disability. The treatment of females with fractures, believe it or not, was to remain under the care of the obstetrician and gynecologist.

I nearly had a fit, but I accepted this as a temporary job with considerable misgiving, not thinking for a moment that I would be working in that center for the next nineteen years, including before long the treatment of fractures in women patients! An additional one of my tasks was to care for British and Indian government servants with musculoskeletal problems. I found myself spending one or two afternoons each week applying plaster of paris jackets to people with low back pain. This, incredible as it sounds, was the accepted treatment in those days for disabling low back pain. The work of applying the jackets was done in a small plaster room with quite inadequate ventilation and a corrugated iron roof with no insulation. It was quite hard physical work, done in tropical heat with the midday sun beating down on that iron roof. I found this work quite a sweat in more ways than one! My patients did not appreciate being encased in plaster for six weeks in our equatorial climate!

About three years later a young British doctor with a London University bachelor of medicine degree and an American diploma in osteopathy arrived in Nairobi. He started a private practice in the town, and his work was mainly in manipulation of the spine and other joints. He was an unusual person who, living in tropical conditions, dressed for work in a navy blue pinstripe suit, drove an ancient Chevrolet, and lived in an old iron bungalow with no water-borne sanitation and a little house down the garden for sanitary purposes.

There is an apocryphal story of the British orthopedic surgeon who flew out to Kenya at the request of this doctor, whose house guest he was, to perform the first lumbar discectomy ever in East Africa. Before dinner on the first evening the surgeon wended his way down the garden to empty his bladder. As he didn't return to the house for twenty minutes, his host went out to find out if all was well. The orthopod, cowering on his throne in the outhouse, complained, "As I came across the lawn I stepped on a bloody great snake, and I'm not leaving here till I know someone has killed it." The host shined his torch back and forth across the grass to discover the garden hose that had been left on the lawn!

This unusual but kindly doctor took pity on me and on the physical therapist who worked with me at that time. He taught us, by modern standards quite inadequately, something about the rudiments of spinal manipulation. Chiropractors and osteopaths would today be shocked to think that people with so little training should be allowed to do this kind of work. There were no government regulations about this and no qualified physician to undertake the work. This was Africa, and I consoled myself with the thought that what the two of us could do was a lot better than nothing! Spinal manipulation under these conditions made all the difference to many patients and opened a door into an exciting new world for the two of us. A great thing for me, I no longer had to sweat in the tropical heat whilst putting on plaster jackets.

At medical school in England I had heard vaguely about the work of osteopaths and chiropractors, usually in terms that were somewhat derogatory. The manipulative treatment given by one of our young London surgeons, a broth of a boy, did not impress me. He manipulated unsuspecting patients with considerable force under a general anesthetic. I never saw any one of them again and so cannot tell if they were helped, were wise enough not to see the surgeon again, or had perhaps passed on to higher service!

But fifty years ago in the far-off tropics patients were satisfied. Quickly I became convinced of the great value of spinal manipulation. I didn't understand the rationale for this kind of approach, any more than I understood the reason for many of the other things I had to do as a young, inexperienced orthopedic surgeon! When visiting in Britain or America I used to say that for many years I was the best orthopedic surgeon between Cairo and Johannesburg, wait for my audience to gasp at my apparent arrogance, then add "because I was the only one!"

Later on I found out that other doctors felt as I did. When it is convenient to do so for one reason or another, orthodox doctors can be rapidly converted to belief in chiropractic and osteopathy and indeed in other kinds of complementary medicine. Looking back I have to admit that we probably were practicing mobilization rather than manipulation, but many patients were helped.

53

When years later I found myself working in a rehabilitation unit on the Canadian prairies, I attempted to introduce the idea of using spinal manipulation as a form of treatment for neck and back pain. I was told in no uncertain terms that this was no task for physical therapists. By chance I discovered a gentleman, Dr. Gordon Potter, a chiropractor who had moved from British Columbia to Brisbane to study for a medical degree. I believe he put himself through medical school by manipulating the spines of the medical teaching staff! Dr. Potter agreed to manipulate the spines of patients I referred to him in his downtown office when we thought this was indicated. This was a most fruitful cooperative effort, to the advantage of both our patients and ourselves.

Dr. Potter introduced me to Dr. Herbert Vear, Dr. Donald Sutherland, and their colleagues at the Canadian Memorial Chiropractic College in Toronto. On first acquaintance I think they were as suspicious of me as I was of them, but surely and slowly we became good friends, much to my advantage and perhaps a bit to theirs. We came eventually to an ever-closer degree of cooperation. This, after a carefully planned start at slow tempo, led to the inauguration of a scheme whereby postgraduate chiropractic students from Toronto spent six to twelve months in Saskatoon. Half of their time was in chiropractic work and half teaching sessions in the departments of orthopedics, rheumatology, neurology, radiology, and the pain clinic in the university hospital. Patients were referred for manipulation to the chiropractic clinic in the town, which was separate from the hospital.

In this setting the students worked toward completing a fellowship in chiropractic clinical sciences from the Canadian Memorial Chiropractic College in Toronto. Some of them obtained master's degrees at the University of Saskatchewan. The final step in this long period of cooperation has been the formation in a downtown office in Saskatoon of an interdisciplinary musculoskeletal clinic for the rehabilitation of severely injured patients who fail to recover from more simple and straightforward medical, chiropractic, or osteopathic forms of treatment. This clinic is managed by a chiropractor, Dr. Dale Mierau, with the help of another chiropractor, an internist, a rheumatologist, a psychologist, a neurologist, physical therapists, exercise therapists, and a surgeon, among others.

It has been very rewarding for me to watch these developments as they have taken place one after the other. I experienced some initial difficulties right at the start from the medical licensing authorities because of my contacts with chiropractors. Early on I had to address the provincial College of Physicians and Surgeons of Saskatchewan on the subject of working with chiropractors and found the members of the council a formidable group! After considerable delay they sanctioned my working with chiropractors under the most stringent conditions. These difficulties, initially somewhat humiliating for the chiropractor, were surmounted without much difficulty and are now past history. Two years after my interview the council changed its thinking and stated that it was in their opinion perfectly ethical for physicians and chiropractors to cooperate.

One amusing incident occurred during a very friendly combined meeting of orthopedic surgeons and chiropractors in London in the 1980s. During this time my wife and I invited a Finnish chiropractor friend to dinner. He turned up with ten friends! Fortunately we were staying at a hotel run by Irish people, among whom the impossible can still happen. Having told us that it would be impossible to accommodate us, the young Irish lady who was manager of the dining room told us to come back in half an hour. A table had been prepared for thirteen, and we had an excellent meal with ninety percent of Finland's chiropractors. This experience reinforced in my mind the importance of combining tact and persistence.

On one occasion at a private dinner the president of the university said, "K-W, I think you're a brave man to work with chiropractors." I replied, "Not brave, sir, just intelligent." I've been rewarded by requests to talk to chiropractors in different countries, by honorary membership in several chiropractic associations, and by an honorary doctor of laws degree from chiropractic colleges in the United States and Canada. More than this, it has been very stimulating to watch developing contacts between physicians in orthodox medicine, chiropractors, osteopaths, and others in an increasing number of clinics in North America and elsewhere.

It has been regrettable that for so long medical physicians have not been officially permitted to refer their patients to chiropractors, or to any other practitioners in complementary or alternative medicine. In British

Columbia the College of Physicians and Surgeons had a written policy stating that its members should not refer patients in this manner, even though the policy seemed never to be strictly enforced. The mere existence of such an edict may well have had deterring influence on some physicians who would otherwise have been prepared to work with those in other disciplines in the integrated management of their patients. We can say now that this is almost a matter of past history. Chiropractic enjoys a high reputation in most circles in the United Kingdom, Europe, Scandinavia, and North America and many M.D.s and D.C.s are working together quite happily to the benefit of themselves and of their patients.

Chiropractic manipulation, as defined by the Swiss chiropractor Dr. Sandoz, is a passive manual maneuver during which a synovial joint is carried suddenly beyond the normal physiological range of movement, without exceeding the boundaries of anatomical integrity. The characteristic is a thrust that is given at the end of the normal passive range of movement, usually accompanied by a cracking sound. Four zones can be distinguished: (1) active range of movement, (2) passive range of movement, (3) movement into the paraphysiological space, and (4) not permitted because it would injure the joint, into the pathological zone. The thrust is of high velocity and low amplitude. This is a skilled procedure.

The effects of manipulation can be explained on the grounds of mechanical and reflex mechanisms. The mechanical are: joint cavitation, increase in range of movement, breaking adhesions, and joint and muscle receptor stimulation. The reflex are: inhibition of pain, relaxation of paraspinal muscles, and stimulation of the autonomic nervous system. The subject of manipulation has been dealt with at length by Mierau and colleagues in the fourth edition of *Managing Low Back Pain*, edited by Kirkaldy -Willis and Bernard (Churchill Livingstone, 1999).

In theory a manipulation has its main effect on a posterior facet joint. There may also be an effect on the multifidus muscle overlying the joint. It is reasonable to assume that the effect is on both joint and muscle. In cases of back pain due to a joint or overlying muscle, relief is obtained from manipulation in eighty to eighty-five percent of cases. In refractory cases relief can be obtained in a further eight to ten percent of patients by injection at a later date of a local anesthetic to the joint and overlying muscle, followed immediately by further manipulation.

It has been these contacts with chiropractors and osteopaths that have led me to an increasing interest in alternative and complementary medicine and to the conviction that this is the right way for the future, both for cost-effectiveness and for much better treatment for our patients. My appreciation of the work of members of the chiropractic profession encourages me to comment frankly on the work of this branch of medicine. There are still chiropractors who think that it is mandatory to manipulate the spine of every patient who comes to see them and to manipulate more than one region of the spine on each visit. Some perhaps do not take time to examine the patient adequately at each visit to be sure there are no complications. This is probably the main reason why legal proceedings are, on occasion, brought against the chiropractor and is in fact the main reason why patients sue their orthodox physician! Another cause of complaint is that some chiropractors proceed to manipulate the spine without first listening to what the patient has to say, and more rarely that they sometimes persist with manipulation without seeking a further opinion when the symptoms do not respond to treatment.

It seems illogical, to say the least, that some cervical spine therapists focus on the two upper cervical vertebrae, whether they are treating low back and leg pain or neck pain and headache. Similarly, craniosacral therapists focus on the upper and lower extremes of the axial skeleton, the cranium, and the sacrum, ignoring the cervical, thoracic, and lumbar areas. I have read much about craniosacral therapy and have attended seminars where this modality was being discussed, but I have to admit that I still do not understand the mechanisms under which it works to relieve pain.

Quantum mechanics discusses the way in which the observer and the observed are linked together. The change that takes place in the subatomic and in the macroscopic realm is still in ghost form, a probability only, until the observer records the result. This means that reality, what happens in the physical world, is dependent on a human observer, a fact difficult to swallow but impossible to ignore. Applying this quantum observation to a modality such as craniosacral therapy, or indeed to any other modality, we reach the conclusion that the attitude of the observer, the physician, to the observed, the patient, and their interaction is more important than the nature of the treatment given.

It is reasonable if not imperative to apply this dictum to conventional and other forms of complementary treatment, as well. In one way this is a humbling thought, but more than that it is very comforting! The importance of the beliefs of the physician is upheld by double-blind studies of 1974 and 1977. One researcher found that vitamin E was significantly more effective than a placebo in treating angina pectoris, but only when the prescribing physician believed in it. Similar experiments in the use of meprobamate as a tranquilizer demonstrated that it was more effective than a placebo, again only when the prescriber believed in its effectiveness. Quantum theory also teaches us that there is more than one way of looking at every problem. I am content to go along with the work of respected colleagues when I don't yet in my ignorance understand what they are doing.

A number of chiropractors espouse the use of manipulation to treat lesions other than musculoskeletal ones. There are two main groups of chiropractors: (1) those who employ manipulation only to treat lesions of the facet joints of the cervical, thoracic, and lumbar spine and of the posterior muscles and other musculoskeletal lesions, in particular those caused by long hours at computer or office desk; (2) those who treat extra spinal lesions, such as otitis media, infantile colic, asthma, and conditions affecting the autonomic nervous system as well as musculoskeletal conditions. There is no difficulty in giving wholehearted support for the former. More double-blind controlled trials have been done on manipulation for spinal lesions than on any other condition. Yet there are doubts in some people's minds about the effects of manipulation for the lesions described under (2), above.

I believe that the most effective chiropractors are those who supplement chiropractic manipulation by other modalities, such as massage, physical therapy, acupuncture, muscle energy techniques, nutrition, and mind/body therapy. I myself have learned a great deal about the treatment of painful lesions in muscles from my chiropractic friends. It is my hope that chiropractic colleges will give more attention to teaching these two things in the future. The value of chiropractic is so great that it would be disastrous if it was lessened because of failure on the part of the chiropractic colleges to give their students adequate instruction in the matters mentioned above.

It goes without saying that we physicians in orthodox medicine are far from being above criticism. We need to pull our socks up. There is much for us to learn from our friends and colleagues in chiropractic and other branches of complementary medicine.

A chiropractor might well say, "Thanks, Dr. K-W, for what you've had to say about your contacts with chiropractors. This is very encouraging for the members of my profession. Personally I would emphasize the value of attention to nutrition and lifestyle management. Can you tell us in a few words what role you think we chiropractors should play?"

My answer would be, "You chiropractors have a very important place in the treatment of many lesions of the musculoskeletal system. Orthopedic surgeons are the right people to treat fractures and major dislocations and other acute injuries. When on occasion an operation is indicated, we are the people to do it. That leaves a high percentage of lesions—the greatest proportion—that are best treated by the chiropractor or osteopath. These lesions of muscle, fascia, ligaments, and joints should, I'm sure, be treated by you people. We should be referring them to you much more often.

Now that so many of us are spending good deal of time each day sitting in front of the computer, minor lesions in muscle, such as the "mouse syndrome," are increasingly common. Many hours at the computer are the cause also of much neck and shoulder pain and stiffness. It is the enthusiastic chiropractor who can do most to help such patients, using simple muscle energy techniques. Attention to nutrition, vitamin therapy, and lifestyle are most important, too." (We'll have more to say about this in another chapter.)

A neurologist might well say, "I've had a lot of help from chiropractors and have been very satisfied with the benefits my patients have got from them, so my questions are not unduly critical. Sometimes I've thought that members of your profession concentrate only on manipulation or what you call "adjustment." I know this modality is very valuable, but I'd like to know if you think that chiropractors should use other methods that you haven't yet mentioned."

The chiropractor might answer, "You're right. Many of us do tend to concentrate on spinal manipulation, sometimes to the neglect of other forms of treatment. We should also be prepared to use soft-tissue techniques, massage, muscle energy techniques, and, if we have had the proper training, acupuncture. It might be good for the chiropractor to incorporate therapeutic touch, relaxation, imaging, and other similar mind/body techniques."

A rheumatologist might comment, "I know that chiropractors don't have as many complications from their work as neurosurgeons or orthopedic surgeons. Some people say that we doctors are good at burying our mistakes! There is however the awkward affair of injury to the vertebral artery that on very rare occasions follows a manipulation of the cervical spine."

To that the chiropractor might answer, "In fifty years of practice I have known personally of two patients who suffered from manipulation of the cervical spine. Both developed a cerebellar thrombosis. One made a complete recovery; the other died. Both had only one vertebral artery. In one of these two instances I thought that the chiropractors concerned had been very thorough in their examination and management. In the other I thought, perhaps wrongly, that the therapists concerned might have exhibited greater care. I know you'll agree that every procedure—medical, surgical, or manipulative—has its own particular complications.

"In dealing with problems affecting the cervical spine, the vertebral artery is a structurally weak link. We need to remember that at the base of the occiput, at C1 and at C2, the artery makes two hairpin bends which must be treated with great respect. It is difficult to see how the manipulator's thrust can injure the artery if the thrust, a high-velocity, low-amplitude procedure, is so planned that the movement between the facets of the cervical vertebrae is no more than one eighth of an inch. I look back to days in chiropractic college and remember what a sweat it was to master the anatomy of the vertebral artery. It was still harder work, much harder, to master the technique of cervical spine manipulation. When something is not quite right after a cervical spine manipulation, the chiropractor should refer the patient at once to a neurologist or other specialist."

Another chiropractor might comment, "Many of us are hesitant to ask the M.D. for help. In the past we have suffered rebuffs. I believe that we could give even better treatment to our patients if we knew we could get the willing help of an orthopedic or neurosurgeon quickly when we thought it advisable. Can anyone here give me some useful advice about this?"

A third chiropractor might add, "Yes, I appreciate your difficulty. When I was newly in practice I had exactly the same problem. Then one day a neurosurgeon referred me a patient. I wrote to thank him for the referral and again when I had treated the patient, who fortunately was relieved of his symptoms. One day, passing his office, I screwed up my courage and went in to see him. He turned out to be a very friendly man. After that he referred more patients to me. Bit by bit we became still better friends. Sometimes we used to have a beer together after office hours. Now we are the best of friends, and that has been a great help both to us and to our patients. Part of our problem is being shy. M.D.s too are shy. I'm sure the secret is to start slowly and gradually learn to have confidence in one another. Nowadays there are many more M.D.s who are friendly than otherwise."

A physical therapist comments, "One of you has mentioned the interdisciplinary center. There's one in our town for the treatment of patients who do not recover quickly after an injury, particularly when it's happened at work. The leader in our center is a chiropractor. I'm fortunate enough to work there. We have two other physical therapists, two other chiropractors, a family doctor, a neurologist, an orthopedic surgeon, a rheumatologist, an occupational therapist, and a psychologist on the staff. We all respect our leader, and we like working together. We have close contact with the CEOs of a number of offices, plants, and factories. When there are difficult family problems in the patient's home, our nurse or someone else on our staff often visits there to check on how things are. When things aren't going well, we always think of the possibility of problems in the workplace or in the home."

It's useful to emphasize the point already made that some chiropractors confine their work to the treatment of the spine and other musculoskeletal lesions, while others believe that conditions affecting the digestive system, allergies, and otitis media in children respond well to chiropractic adjustment. We do not yet have a definitive answer to these matters. From quantum we learn that all the systems in our bodies are closely interrelated. While bearing in mind the possibility that manipulation can help these extraspinal conditions, it seems wise not to form a definite decision till we have more scientific information about this question. Hence the need for rigorous research in this area.

Recently chiropractic has been under attack in reputable journals such as the *New England Journal of Medicine* and the *British Medical Journal*. From the viewpoint of those interested in cooperation between mainstream and complementary medicine, the comments in the *BMJ* appear to paint an unduly cynical picture of the ineffectiveness of spinal manipulation. One can only conclude that those responsible for the attacks are afraid that chiropractic, among other forms of alternative medicine, is poised for great acclaim, and that this will erode the influence of their own disciplines.

There has also been controversy as to the relative value of therapeutic touch and chiropractic manipulation in the treatment of asthma. It is now necessary that chiropractors and others in manual therapy demonstrate scientifically that they can produce better results than those employing other kinds of hands on therapy.

I (WHK-W) consider myself very fortunate to have had the help of a friendly MD Manual Therapist early on and the help of a MD chiropractor later on. For many years now I've had as many friends who are chiropractors as MD s. You people have taught me so much and I'd be quite lost without your help". I can go as far as to say that my contacts with chiropractors and others has made the practice of medicine much more enjoyable for me and much more profitable for my patients. It's good to think that this happy state of affairs is going to be widespread throughout the world and regarded as normal in days to come.

I picked up some knowledge about the history of chiropractic long after I was convinced that it was a valuable form of therapy. So in this chapter I've left the historical details till the end. Andrew Still, the founder of osteopathy, put forward his new ideas about spinal manipulation in 1874. D.D. Palmer, an itinerant tradesman and later school teacher, published his first notes and papers in a few years later. Both names are closely connected in discussions on manipulation.

D.D. Palmer began his chiropractic work in Davenport, Iowa, working to establish a school there in 1895. By 1902 he had only produced 15 graduates. He was a controversial figure who offended his colleagues by his satire and by his controversial manner. For all this the colleagues were undoubtedly impressed. He placed great emphasis on what he called the subluxation, a mal-alignment of one vertebra on another. In later years he left Davenport and traveled to teach in Oregon and California. He returned to Davenport in 1913, a man who'd made important discoveries that had not really gained acceptance. Shortly after this he was killed in an accident.

He was succeeded by his son B.J. Palmer, a teacher of great charisma combined with a tyrannical nature that expressed itself in ruthless opposition to his opponents. Those who met him in his early years said they'd encountered a religious type of experience. He was a brilliant organizer with a striking appearance who dominated the chiropractic scene from 1924 till 1961. He was the titular head. He expanded the osteological laboratory and museum which was started by his father. The A.M.A. council on medical education in 1928 declared that the museum housed the best ever collection of spines. The x-ray department, started only thirteen years after Roentgen, was among the best in the country. The clinic B.J. developed had a full medical and nursing staff with a complete diagnostic laboratory and department of physical medicine. He stated his determination "to sell, serve, and save chiropractic if it took him twenty lifetimes to do it!"

The next generation of broad scope chiropractic spokesmen thought B.J. had forfeited the right of leadership and embraced the difficult task of raising chiropractic to a level where it would be treated seriously in academic circles. At this point chiropractic was lagging behind osteopathy in standards, equipment, teaching staff and clinical work. A chiropractic spokesman in 1917 expressed the opinion that "chiropractic students should not be wasting their time on chemistry, bacteriology and the like but concentrating on palpation and adjustment." It was not surprising that the standing of chiropractic was at a low ebb.

In 1924 there were few chiropractic schools that gave the student more than eighteen months education, without any teaching of chemistry, physics, bacteriology or microscopy. The emphasis was all on acquiring the art of spinal adjustment. In 1930 an exam in basic science was introduced for all students of medicine. The pass rate for MD students was about eighty percent and that for chiropractic students twenty-two percent! The standing of chiropractors fell dramatically. Chiropractic sought alliances with other disciplines such as Naturopathy and Homeopathy. After World War II the standing of chiropractic fell again but fortunately there was an upswing about 1946.

Dr. John Nugent and other chiropractic teachers worked hard to enhance the position of their discipline with considerable success. The profession had no public funding but in spite of this by 1950 the enrolment of chiropractic students had greatly increased in all the schools with a two year preclinical course of teaching in basic science and a four year clinical course. The standard of teaching was almost comparable to that in orthodox schools. Dr. Nugent became known as the Flexner of Chiropractic.

Chiropractors suffered considerably on and off between 1904 and 1950. In New York in 1922 more than one hundred chiropractors were arrested for practicing without a license. In 1925 the A.M.A. apparently decided to seek an early end to chiropractic, chiefly to do away with an unwanted competitor. In the chapter on Mainstream Medicine we discussed the fierce combat between the A.M.A. and the chiropractic profession. A few outstandingly determined courageous leaders of chiropractic, aided and guided by a very able tenacious lawyer, defeated the A.M.A. in the supreme court. We bear in mind that the latter sought to demolish chiropractic, partly thinking it an inferior profession and no doubt also to eliminate competition and preserve their position of supremacy.

Chiropractors can now hold up their heads. In many countries today patient visits to chiropractors and others in alternative medicine equal or even exceed those to physicians in orthodox medicine. As we look back to the early days when D.D. Palmer was pioneering the new specialty at the beginning of the century, picture in our minds the struggle that he and his successors were engaged in and realize how much new ground they had to cover, it is almost unbelievable to think that so much has been achieved in less than one hundred years.

In chiropractic, as also in homeopathy, osteopathy and naturopathy, we can detect the two strands that are essential for the success of any worthwhile healing venture, the 'idea-stuff' and the 'physical matter-stuff.' As we saw earlier these are a vital part of what quantum theory teaches. Put another way, the philosophy propounded by chiropractic teaches us first that the aim is for patients to know that they can heal themselves, a vitalist life-force. In the second place is the emphasis on the physical aspect, that chiropractors adjust the spine by hand only. In this materialistic age it is difficult for orthodox conventional medicine to appreciate such an holistic approach. This is a lesson that I and my colleagues have to learn.

# — 7 —

# Osteopathy

WE DISCUSSED SOME ASPECTS of osteopathic medicine in our last chapter which dealt mainly with chiropractic. There is much more to be said about this important branch of medicine. It is difficult to determine whether this discipline stands on its own, as a branch of mainstream medicine or whether it is complementary. Perhaps it's better to think of it as both of these. Osteopathy has its roots like many other kinds of modern medicine in the developments in China, India and Greece. We have discussed these elsewhere and will attempt now to trace its growth in modern times during the last century.

As a boy I (WHK-W) remember being intrigued by the story of another boy in North Wales, Hugh Owen Thomas, whose uncle was a bonesetter. He used to take Hugh with him in his pony-trap when making his rounds to see his patients from to farm in the delightful countryside of North Wales. That was in the last part of the nineteenth century. As they jogged along the narrow winding roads the uncle would take one bone or another, such as a carpal scaphoid or metacarpal, out of his pocket and get Hugh to tell him the name and side of the bone, without looking, just by feeling. It took a while but Hugh became expert in what was to begin with for him no more than an amusing guessing game. The youngster became so intrigued that eventually he decided to be a doctor, studied for this at Liverpool University, and eventually qualified with a Bachelor of Medicine degree.

His experiences with the uncle led him to start practice in what is now orthopedic surgery, at a time before there were any orthopedic surgeons in Britain. Liverpool was a busy city and port, and many of its citizens were poor and undernourished. Tuberculosis was rampant. There were no hospital beds for the treatment of tuberculous bones and joints. Hugh ran his practice in a large house he'd acquired and began to treat people with TB of spine, hip, and knee as resident patients, using frames and splints of metal and leather, padded rather poorly and very uncomfortable: all this to rest the affected joint in the correct position.

He began to get good results and soon acquired a great reputation. The man who constantly wore a sea captain's cap was always welcome in the slums of the great city. It rested with his successor, Robert Jones, to refine the treatment Hugh had pioneered and make the splints more comfortable. In Britain orthopedics had its origin in the work of an unorthodox Welsh bonesetter. In North America orthopedic advances took place in a very similar manner. It's not really surprising that the mainstream owes much to the unorthodox.

Osteopathic medicine is in a unique position among the stars of orthodox and complementary medicine. Hippocrates, father of modern medicine, used manipulative techniques, assisted by his brother in the gymnasium by the harbor in Cos. In the nineteenth century Edward Harrison, moving from Edinburgh to London, employed manual procedures. The eminent physician James Paget, writing in British medical journals with an open mind, applauded the work of what he thought of as unorthodox bonesetters, It was the American engineer and orthodox medical doctor Andrew Still who, disenchanted with the medical practice of his time at the end of the nineteenth century, formulated a new philosophy that he called osteopathic medicine. That he suffered personally from orthodox treatment did not endear this therapy to him! He gained support both from Oliver Wendell Holmes of Harvard and from Sir William Osler, then Regius Professor of Medicine at Oxford. In 1864 Still lost three children to a meningitis epidemic despite heroic efforts to save them. This led him to reject orthodox medicine and develop ever-greater interest in alternative methods of healing.

D.D. Palmer was a contemporary of Andrew Still. Palmer was not a doctor of medicine but a grocer. He, Palmer, founded chiropractic colleges in Davenport, Iowa and in Oklahoma City during the last decade of the nineteenth century. In those early days there must have been a good deal of overlap between the two disciplines though chiropractic did not profess to be a total school of medicine. Still's early attempts to interest his medical colleagues in his concepts were rebuffed. But before long he became clinically successful and well known throughout the United States and abroad. He attracted many students who came to study his principles, both from North America and elsewhere in the world.

Still assembled a number of key principles in what he considered to be a philosophy, a science, and an art:

(1) The body is a unit: the person is a unit of body, mind, and spirit.
(2) The body is capable of self-regulation, self-healing, and health maintenance.
(3) Structure and function are closely interrelated.
(4) Rational treatment is based upon an understanding of the basic principles of body unity, self-regulation and the interrelationship of structure and function.

At the time these ideas were considered to be heretical though now few would take exception to them. Dr. Philip Greenman writes "In the application of the basic principle of the interrelationship of structure and function Dr. Still developed a system of structural diagnosis of the musculoskeletal system within the context of total patient evaluation, and developed multiple manual medicine procedures designed toward enhancing the functional capacity of the musculoskeletal system, and thus enhance the efficiency of the whole body. The osteopathic profession continues to be recognized for its expertise in the area of structural diagnosis and manual medicine procedures." It sounds as though the musculoskeletal system was the main and most important part of osteopathy with others systems in a position of minor import.

Grounded as he was in the mechanical principles of engineering and those of conventional medicine in the nineteenth century Still constructed a system that was a combination of these and a philosophy and art that he invented himself. The engineering principles started off in a mechanical scientific way but became, as they advanced, confused by the addition of intuitive and philosophical concepts. To say this is not to condemn osteopathy out of hand for at the present time, largely due to the dicta of quantum mechanics, conventional medicine can no longer escape from the accusation that it is influenced by phenomena that are distinctly not scientific. And all the better for that!

During this Twentieth century both osteopaths and some members of the medical profession have been increasingly interested in Manual Medicine. Under the influence of the two Mennells and of the two Cyriaxs, in each case father and son, all four doctors of medicine, the scope of Manual Medicine, and with it of osteopathy, has grown considerably.

Manual medicine came to include: (1)soft tissue therapy, chiefly of muscle, fascia, and joint capsule, (2) mobilization without impulse, (3) muscle energy techniques, (4) mobilization with impulse (manipulation by the chiropractor), (5) indirect techniques, (6) myofascial release (7) craniosacral techniques.

It is difficult for the uninitiated to understand the ins and outs of craniosacral therapy. The fact that well known universally trusted osteopaths like Phillip Greenman accept it inclines me and others to accept it too. Today's physicists accept a quantum finding if they discover that it works in practice, whether they understand it or not. The same goes for modern medicine. We accept a new discovery if and when we find that it works. Of course it's good to know how something works though we medical people tend to produce a tentative answer before we've really tested it to see if it's really true or not.

To begin with there was considerable rivalry between the so called orthodox medicine and osteopathy, partly from fear of something new and partly from financial competition. For many years the orthodox establishment conducted a running battle with both osteopathy and chiropractic. During the middle years of this century there was a rapprochement between those practicing orthodox medicine and those in osteopathy. Critics say that the osteopaths bought peace by accepting the fundamental principles of mainstream medicine as supported by the A.M.A. whilst continuing to practice their own art. The result of this was that osteopathic colleges became equivalent to orthodox medical colleges and the degree of Doctor of Osteopathy (D.O.) equivalent to the degree of Doctor of Medicine (M.D.).

This remarkable *volte-face* gradually led to a situation in which both the M.D. and the D.O. practiced the same type of medicine, almost entirely that of the orthodox style. In many cases the new kind of D.O. appeared to lose interest in manual medicine. The number of osteopaths who practised osteopathy decreased considerably, probably to the advantage of chiropractic. Throughout the United States there are now strong groups of osteopaths who practise manual medicine, often with M.D. colleagues who also limit their practice to manual medicine.

Here then we have a situation in which D.O.s can if they wish engage in both orthodox medicine and the discipline of osteopathy. I have a good friend who graduated from an osteopathic college with a D.O. degree, was a resident in an orthopedic program, and is now professor and head of a well known orthopedic department on the Eastern Sea Board. I don't believe he practices osteopathic medicine though his wife is a chiropractor."

About forty years ago while I (WHK-W) was an orthopedic surgeon in East Africa, I had a cry for help by airmail from an old college friend who had been ordained in the Church of England and had risen to become an archdeacon. He had suffered for months from a very painful shoulder and was eventually referred to an orthopedic surgeon who booked him into hospital for an operation, I think an acromionectomy. In the interim the surgeon went on holiday to Spain, had a heart attack, and died. My friend wrote in some dismay to ask me what he should do now. My young son had a friend who was an osteopath in North London. I got his address and sent it to my friend the archdeacon, recommending strongly that he go to see the osteopath.

It took weeks for my friend to screw up his courage to follow my advice. When the archdeacon got to the osteopath's office, he found that the great man was unable to see him, so he had to opt for an assistant, who manipulated the shoulder on two occasions and cured him. I suspect the problem was a muscle syndrome and not an acromion impingement at all. It was months before my friend, in his next Christmas letter, could bring himself to write and thank me! I laughed and laughed. All's well that ends well. My college friend, his shoulder healed, became a bishop!

It's an advantage for an M.D. who is interested in manual medicine to be able to work with a D.O. who shares the same interest. In fact the M.D. and the D.O. get on very well together. Their common interest is now a very great help. A friend of mine aged about sixty was diagnosed as having angina. He was quite concerned. By chance he was introduced to an M.D., his wife's cousin, who worked closely with osteopaths.

This physician examined my friend and came to the conclusion that the symptoms were due not to angina but to an upper thoracic facet syndrome. Two or three sessions to treat the syndrome completely relieved my friend's symptoms and to his great delight he was back to playing golf. Twenty years later he's still playing golf and is a globe-trotter as well! There is no doubt in my mind that cooperation between the M.D. and the D.O. helps both physicians and the patient. This goes for the D.C. as well in many cases.

Dr. Janet Travell personal physician to President John Kennedy, was an M.D. who worked closely with osteopaths. Her work on myofascial syndromes has revolutionized our ideas about muscle pain. Her approach was a gentle careful one. Great physicians often have some idiosyncrasy. Hers was to wear a shawl over one shoulder. This kept on falling down to be replaced by a characteristic hitching of the shoulder. The onlooker felt that this was an essential part of the maneuvre!

I think osteopaths would agree with the results of experiments done at the University of Ohio. Scientists working in the lab there divided rabbits into five or six groups of a dozen each. The lab assistants fed them all a high-fat diet calculated to give them atherosclerosis of the coronary arteries. They sacrificed all the animals at the end of three months. All of them had developed marked degenerative changes in the arteries, except for those in one group, whose arteries were almost normal.

The mystery was solved when the scientists discovered that the one group of normal animals had been under the care of an assistant who fed his rabbits with great personal attention, stroking them and playing with them in the process. The conclusion—that giving the animals this attention prevented the formation of atherosclerotic plaques in the walls of the arteries. The "little nudges" we mentioned in talking about quantum mechanics made all the difference.

A friend of mine developed, as a teenager, severe pain in the center of his abdomen, accompanied by vomiting. The doctor said he'd got appendicitis and planned his admission to hospital for an operation. The mother was an unusual kind of person. She believed in osteopathy! She told the doctor she'd get back to him shortly and in the meantime took her son to see her osteopath who manipulated my friend's back and abdomen. This completely relieved all the symptoms and signs. Back went mother and son to the family doctor's office. The doctor examined the youngster carefully and was quite flabbergasted to discover that there was no longer any indication of appendicitis. He couldn't approve of what the mother had done but had to admit that he was defeated. This is the story my friend told me some years later.

Now here's the burning question. Was the family doctor wrong in his initial diagnosis? Perhaps the young fellow had been eating green apples? Was this a case of a spontaneous recovery? Or had the manipulation something to do with this very satisfactory result? The appendix is a blind tube with only one opening from the caecum. One possible cause of inflammation of this little organ is that it becomes kinked for some reason or other so that the entrance from the large intestine becomes blocked and then fluid accumulates inside the tube which is stagnant and soon becomes infected.

It's feasible that the manipulation somehow or other reduced the kink so that the opening was again patent and the inflammation subsided.

We'll never know for certain. The condition we call volvulus of the small or large intestine is a kinking and twisting of the gut for no known reason. If left untreated it becomes infected and gangrenous. Another similar example is torsion of the testis. In any case all this makes one think. I call to mind that Still himself undertook visceral manipulation.

My nurse read what I'd written and said "I've read about this debate with great interest. I've been at seminars when one could look round the room and note the number of nods of approval and see that our individual opinions are changing. The simple fact that people representing the old and the new ways of managing disease can sit down together as equals to discuss all these complex problems does I believe more than anything else to help usher in the new approach that in our hearts we all long for. The new paradigm asks for:

(1) emphasis on preventive measures all along the line,
(2) when preventive measures have failed emphasis should be on simple measures of treatment,
(3) only when these have failed should there be recourse to complicated technologies.

A surgeon friend made a comment as he thanked me for letting him in on what he called "these fascinating discussions" which he said were proving an eye opener for him. He went on to say "Most of what you've been discussing is completely new to me. I'm keeping what I hope is an open mind about the relationship between the orthodox and the complementary. All I can say at the moment is that I'm extremely interested. I'd like to think that I might feel able to accept what most of you are advocating. Let's keep in touch. This of course is the attitude of mind that we look for in doing all we can to foster increased cooperation between the disciplines.

# – 8 –

# Physical Therapy

PHYSICAL THERAPY VARIES from practitioner to practitioner, context to context, and often overlaps in methods with osteopathy, chiropractic, and massage. Physical therapy employs manual methods for superficial and deep massage, exercises to build up weak muscles, and stretching to relax tight and contracted soft tissues. It also employs heat, cold, and electrical therapy. It is often applied in a rehabilitative context or to prevent degeneration during prolonged inactivity, either from other forms of therapy or from conditions like poliomyelitis or stroke.

Some physical therapists now "manipulate" joints in the neck, back, and elsewhere, but chiropractors say their own "manipulation" is different from the physical therapist's treatment, which is a "mobilization." Many chiropractors and osteopaths place more emphasis on muscle energy techniques, while many physical therapists emphasize massage and heat, cold, and electrical modalities. Here again, there is some inevitable confusion, because the whole picture is constantly changing and because chiropractors, osteopaths, physical therapists, and other medical practitioners are beginning to work together in offices and hospitals. In spite of the confusion about definition, this is a situation that we would encourage and which we hope will soon become the norm.

As with so many medical modalities, both in today's mainstream and outside it, something like physical therapy first appeared in the West in ancient Greece. We know that Hippocrates and his assistants used the equivalent of physical therapy in the gymnasium in the compound neighboring the harbor at Cos. There must have been other even earlier physicians from whom they inherited such treatments.

In ancient Greece exercise was always an important part of treatment. We have reason to believe that they used traction and spinal manipulation as well. In the temple of Aphrodite at Corinth there were at one point some thousand sacred prostitutes. These people were not there just to provide sex as therapy but also to lead the singing and dancing, which were considered important in healing. In our view, sex is indeed a great God-given healer, though today we don't think its correct and most effective form is between a man and a prostitute but between a husband and wife.

Over the centuries the arsenal of folk medicine generally included massage and similar physical treatments, provided by country people such as farmers. It is rumored that a highly recommended treatment for lumbago and sciatica among country folk was to put the unfortunate sufferer on his face on the kitchen table, cover his back with a large piece of brown paper, and apply a hot iron up and down till the patient cried out, at which time he was pronounced cured! Into what category can we place this novel form of treatment if not that of physical therapy?

In 1825 a French physician, Jacques Delpech, purchased land outside Montpellier in the south of France and built an orthopedic institute in the grounds. Patients with spinal deformities lived there for one to two years while participating in his program of exercises and gymnastics. They were dressed for this in garments rather like leotards, and Delpech required them to perform the most incredible contortions on ropes and swings.

One wonders at the stamina that enabled these patients to stay the course for so long a time. This experiment has been described as one of the first attempts to form a "back school," something quite common today. We do not know if Delpech's institute ever reached its goals, for in

1832 Delpech himself was shot and killed by a deranged patient. Could it be that the prolonged and arduous regime of treatment had anything to do with the onset of this derangement?

In the early years of the twentieth century a form of massage was developed in Sweden known today simply as Swedish massage. A system of "spine education" was developed in association with it. This practice spread to other European countries, arriving in the United Kingdom rather later in the twentieth century. In 1957 a similar program had been initiated in Sydney, Australia. It would seem that in Europe the discipline of physical therapy has developed from Swedish massage and spread from that continent to the United Kingdom. Developments in physical therapy at the orthopedic center at Oswestry in England early in the twentieth century exerted considerable influence on what in Britain is called "physiotherapy." One of the first British schools to teach physiotherapy was opened in Oswestry.

For me (WHK-W) the introduction to physical therapy was such a happy one that from that time in 1944 until the present time I've always enjoyed working with physical therapists. I owe a great deal in particular to two British physical therapists with whom I worked in Nairobi when employed by the government of Kenya. The first, Frank Keer Keer, was brilliant and unorthodox. I wasn't too impressed with the equipment he used, such as short-wave diathermy and ultrasound machines, but when it came to helping me treat African patients with tuberculous spines and hips, post-poliomyelitis contractures, and other problems like those, he was magnificent.

Part of the treatment for these conditions before the advent of anti-tuberculous drugs was to have the patient lie at rest in a plaster shell for months. Rest to the affected joint, and to the whole patient too, was the order of the day. In most cases, as soon as the patient was fit enough, I did a fusion, a bone grafting operation, and kept the patient inert and in plaster for a full three more months.

Ordinarily, the well-being of anyone, healthy or ill, depends on the maintenance of activity and movement. But with tuberculous patients, the need for immobility took precedence. When Frank Keer Keer suggested group exercise for fifteen minutes twice a day for the patients lying in their shells and plasters out in the garden, I was shaken. This was contrary to the accepted treatment in the 1940s. But fortunately I accepted his advice. He supervised, cajoled, and encouraged our patients to use their healthy joints and muscles vigorously, with much waving of his arms and wagging of his tongue. They seemed to enjoy the process, which was accompanied by a good deal of laughter. To my surprise and delight they all did extremely well, and their recovery was more rapid than I'd expected.

In the end I became a willing convert to this new therapy of "health through activity." Over the years I have used this method for the management of fractures, dislocations, and other orthopedic conditions with great success. A visiting professor of preventive medicine from Newcastle University in the north of England commented, "But this is preventive surgery!" All this I owe to my unconventional colleague.

I am also much indebted to another British physiotherapist, Winifred Cannell, who came to us later on from Oswestry in the north of England, where orthopedic pioneering for the whole of Britain took place under Dame Agnes Hunt and Sir Robert Jones at the beginning of the twentieth century. Winifred introduced me to a new way of treating fractures of the bones of the leg—the femur and tibia. This was Perkins' Traction, invented by George Perkins, professor of surgery at St. Thomas Hospital in London. The apparatus he used for the treatment of these fractures, with traction on cords attached to a pin through the femur or tibia, was simple to construct, easy to set up, cheap, and very effective. The patient was able to move the joints by using the muscles of the legs, all the time that the fracture was healing, and so avoid the complications of stiff joints and atrophied muscles. I see the work of physical therapists today in the light of what those two taught me many years ago.

Let us take a look here at the variety of ways in which physical therapists approach their work. These depend on the attitude of the therapist and the diversity of the tasks confronting them. Physical Therapists see a great variety of patients, and their work is quite diverse. The rapport between physical therapist and patient is very important. In all disciplines there are some pitfalls.

Some P.T.s are concerned primarily with increasing muscle strength. Muscle strength is important in rehabilitation but not exclusively so. Flexibility and the range of joint movement are also very important. Too much emphasis on increasing muscle strength tends to make the therapist expect patients to exert themselves as much as or more than they possibly can. This may involve more than the patient can give, to his or her detriment.

On the other hand, some physical therapists are inclined to depend almost exclusively on technically assisted modalities, like short-wave diathermy or the application of heat, cold, and ultrasound. Ice and heat are very important methods of treatment but need to be supplemented by other modalities, particularly those that encourage patients to make an effort to contribute to their own recovery. Too much effort can be harmful, but exercises are especially important to restore strength to weakened muscles.

There are physical therapists who are concerned primarily with the mobilization of stiff and painful joints and, like chiropractors and osteopaths, with the application of muscle energy techniques, using muscle activity to increase pain free joint movement.

Physical therapists who work in multidisciplinary clinics need all the approaches listed above. The rehabilitation of the injured worker has enlarged the scope of the work done by the physical therapist, often with the help of an occupational therapist and exercise physiologist. Sometimes they work for a Workers' Compensation Board or similar organization. Some therapists include a work-hardening gymnasium in their office setup, a very important addition. Some physical and occupational therapists work in a factory or plant to help facilitate the return to work of the injured worker.

All these have added considerably to the scope of the therapist, now much enlarged to include sports medicine, a fascinating and specialized branch of the work. Working in these contexts calls for much patience and persistence. The therapist often has to deal with problems beyond issues of physical rehabilitation and must cultivate the ability to work with other physical therapists, occupational therapists, and psychologists. The best results are obtained when orthodox physicians, physical therapists, and practitioners of alternative and complementary medicine learn how to cooperate better with one another and how to appreciate working together.

In sum, there are many different kinds of physical therapists, and the tasks they have to tackle are very diverse. A well-trained, skilled, patient, and perceptive physical therapist is worth his or her weight in gold. The relationship between any physician and patient is of great importance. The same applies to physical therapist and patient. This is sometimes difficult to achieve in a clinic where a number of therapists are working together, but a skillful and understanding clinic director will be sensitive to issues of rapport between therapist and patient.

We haven't gone into any great detail but have tried to give you a sense of the situations under which physical therapists work. Orthodox physicians, physical therapists, and practitioners in alternative and complementary medicine are striving to learn how to cooperate with one another better and how to appreciate and enjoy working with each other. We could call it a team approach, or better still a quantum approach, because the members of the four groups—medical, osteopathic, chiropractic, and physiotherapeutic—already complement one another's work. We feel certain that this cooperation is on the increase in a most satisfactory way.

# — 9 —

# Chinese Medicine, Acupuncture, and Herbal Medicine

WE WOULD LIKE TO BEGIN our discussion of Chinese medicine, acupuncture, and herbal medicine with a discussion between an advocate of Chinese medicine and a Western orthodox doctor. Then we will add some comments of our own and go on to say something about the role of herbal medicine.

*Western Doctor:* Could you tell me what are the main characteristics of Traditional Chinese Medicine?

*Chinese Doctor:* Traditional Chinese Medicine emphasizes prevention rather than cure. Chinese people pay us to keep them fit rather than for help when they are ill. We recommend measures that increase internal resistance to disease and treat the individual as a whole, mind and body together as one entity. We have discovered many natural substances, mainly natural products like herbs, that have tonic effects on the tissues and that protect against disease, whether it comes from outside or inside the body.

A notable example is gingko, native to both China and Japan, which is effective for circulatory disorders and helps to improve mental faculties. It has recently become popular among acupuncturists and is perhaps the best-known herb used by TCM in the West. It is used to rectify imbalances that have not yet become what one might consider the symptom of a disease.

*Western Doctor:* What exactly is acupuncture?

*Chinese Doctor:* It is the application of needles to specific points on the surface of the body to influence the flow of energy.

*Western Doctor:* Is it true that acupuncture can be used as an anesthetic?

*Chinese Doctor:* Oh yes. Even major operations such as open-heart surgery can be performed under acupuncture anesthesia. This has been verified by a number of physicians from the West, who on visits to China have been present at major operations performed in this way. Westerners find it quite uncanny to see a conscious, smiling young lady, lying on the operating table, her chest draped with sterile towels and her heart exposed through a large thoracic incision.

In spite of the efficacy of acupuncture, however, in China at the present time the majority of operative procedures are performed using Western anesthetic methods. In China, Western-style medicine exists alongside of TCM. In fact, there are basically three different forms of orthodox medical practice in China today: TCM, Western medicine, and a certain development of TCM that uses Western technology to extend its power. For instance, there is a new form of acupuncture that uses needles that conduct electric currents.

*Western Doctor:* Could you tell me something about the basic principles of TCM?

*Chinese Doctor:* The basic tenet of Traditional Chinese Medicine is the existence of *qi* (ch'i), the life force. This manifests itself in two opposite but complementary characters, *yin* and *yang*. The yin and yang represent pairs of qualities such as dark and light, receptive and active, female and male, and cold and hot. Yin and yang interact to produce the normal function of the body. Qi flows along fourteen invisible channels, the meridians, which crisscross head, arms, legs, and trunk, and pass deep within all the tissues. These channels surface at 360 acupuncture "points." Each meridian services one or more specified organs, such as heart, kidney, liver, and so on. The organs (or organ systems) can be influenced by stimulating the appropriate acupuncture points.

Many things can alter the flow of qi, such as diet, hard work, cancer, infection, stress, as well as environmental conditions such as wind, cold, fire, and dampness. These factors cause an imbalance of the yin and yang, which in turn causes illness. Correct stimulation of acupuncture points can rectify the imbalance and restore the normal flow of qi. Excess of yang—too much exposure to heat for instance—leads to a disorder of the yin. Excess of yin—too much exposure to the cold—leads to a disorder of yang.

According to TCM there are in the body five *zang*, or solid organs: the heart, lungs, spleen, liver, and kidneys; and six *fu*, or hollow organs: the gall bladder, stomach, small intestine, large intestine, bladder, and the mysterious *ti-jiac* organ that is situated near the pericardium. To each organ is connected a meridian, extending from the physical organ in the body cavity up to the surface of the body and terminating either in the hand or the foot.

What TCM means by the "organs" is not quite the same as the organs with same name in Western medicine. For TCM the organ includes the meridian systems associated with it, emotional and spiritual factors that are also linked to it, as well as certain other factors. The kidneys, for instance, are associated with the emotion of fear and also function to store qi.

*Western Doctor:* How do you know that qi, the meridians, and the yin and yang exist?

*Chinese Doctor:* Westerners often find it difficult to accept theoretical concepts like qi, yin and yang, or the meridians, since direct observation of the kind that can be accomplished through the use of instruments such as the microscope or by biochemical tests cannot reveal their existence. But the observation of these forces and systems does, we believe, occur through a very special kind of attention that we are trained to apply. We know, for instance, how to observe changes in the color and texture of the tongue and skin and to detect nuances in the qualities of the pulses along the meridians. These observations allow us to perceive the state of a person's qi. We know that what we observe in this way corresponds to the patient's complaints, and we know that applying appropriate herbs, acupuncture needling, or specific exercises or meditation practices changes what we observe and relieves the patient's symptoms.

In China we have found over a long period of time that the concepts that our wise men and women have enunciated help us to prevent and cure disease. We are prepared to modify our concepts in the light of further knowledge, but we have found over several thousand years of observation and practice that these ideas are broad enough to allow us to assimilate whatever new information we are able to gather.

We do not have a theory of the mechanism of how these processes work in a material, Western sense. But you Westerners have to remember that you yourselves use many drugs without understanding why or how they work. Aspirin is a notable example. The Babylonians noticed more than three thousand years ago that infusions of the bark of the willow tree were effective in alleviating pain and in treating fever. Toward the end of the nineteenth century, chemists at the Bayer factory in Germany discovered the chemical composition of the active component of the bark, salicylic acid, and then worked out how to manufacture a more active product: acetylsalicylic acid. This is the most commonly used of all your drugs, but no one knows how it actually relieves pain or reduces fever. You accept it because you have observed that it works.

Another example: your quantum theory has led to more important technological advances than any other theory in modern science, yet no physicist understands how quantum theory works. You accept it because of the far-reaching, useful discoveries that result from its application. I ask you to accept Traditional Chinese Medicine and its techniques of acupuncture and its application of herbs in a similar spirit.

*Western Doctor:* You mentioned that TCM uses the observation of pulses in diagnosis. Could you tell me something about this?

*Chinese Doctor:* TCM places great emphasis on a detailed examination of the pulse at the wrist. Nine pulses are postulated at each wrist, each with as many as 27 differentiable characteristics: weak or strong, shallow or deep, for example. Each organ system has its distinctive pulse.

Pulse diagnosis is combined with other observations including emotional factors, personal preferences (such as a preference for cold drinks or hot drinks), and patterns of sleep, to form a series of well-defined syndromes.

The syndromes are then understood in terms of yin and yang deficiency and excess and in relation to specific organ systems. Acupuncture is then applied to the appropriate meridians in combination with herbs, massage, exercise, and/or meditation to relieve the syndrome. You can see that this way of combining physical symptoms with emotional and preference patterns is a very holistic approach to medicine.

*Western Doctor:* Getting back to acupuncture. Can you say something more about the specific procedures used?

*Chinese Doctor:* Well, when a needle is inserted, the patient feels something like a mosquito bite rather than a sensation of pain. The needles used in acupuncture are hair thin and vary in length from one to several inches. Up to twelve needles are used at a session, twirled and left in place for varying lengths of time.

Besides diagnosis by syndromes, some specific symptoms can be treated by needling specific acupuncture points. There are thus specific points to relieve headache, to bring one round to consciousness after a faint, for relieving nausea, etc. There are also specific combinations of points that work for certain conditions. For low back pain needles are placed in points along meridians in the leg, hand, and ear. For circulatory problems they may be placed in the fifth toe.

Sometimes other means besides needles are used to stimulate the points: moxibustion, for instance, is the practice of burning certain herbs over the points. Sometimes acupressure, the application of pressure with the fingers, is used. The patient can learn to apply acupressure to him or herself, and you will often see Chinese and other Asian people, during idle moments, performing acupressure on their own hands or fingers.

*Western Doctor:* You said that no one has ever demonstrated the existence, of the meridians or how they in fact function. Are there any hypotheses being put forward by Western researchers today about these matters?

*Chinese Doctor:* There are several. Some physicians believe that the effects of acupuncture are basically placebo effects, but this seems inherently implausible in the case of the use of acupuncture for anesthesia during surgical operations. Some physicians are of the opinion that needling by acupuncture causes the release of endorphins, relieving pain in the same way that narcotics do. It has been observed that at the various acupuncture points there are many more subdermal nerve endings than elsewhere, and that more electromagnetic energy is concentrated at the characteristic acupuncture points. It is possible, therefore, that the meridians have something to do with the flow of neuroelectric currents. It has also been hypothesized that the meridians may represent patterns of the flow of piezoelectric currents in the connective tissue.

In the United States acupuncture is a modality that is recognized in the majority of states. There are about three thousand therapists who treat approximately ten million patients a year, but being an acupuncturist is no sinecure. In some states only an M.D. is allowed to use acupuncture; in others, a license can be obtained after attending a quite lengthy and arduous course of instruction, followed by an examination.

From the point of view of Western medical science, the results of acupuncture have been anecdotal for the most part, though there have been several controlled studies on treatment for pain management, for asthma, for drug and alcohol abuse, and for rehabilitation in patients who have had strokes. Rehabilitation has been found effective, particularly if applied soon after a stroke. Acupuncture is of help for gastrointestinal disorders that have resisted conventional treatment, for relief of pain after surgery, to prevent or reduce nausea during chemotherapy, and in pain clinics. An important practical point: great care must betaken not to use infected needles because of the danger of AIDS and other infectious diseases.

# Plants, Herbs, and Drugs

We would like to conclude this chapter with a brief discussion of herbal medicine, both as an aspect of Chinese medicine, and as alternative medicine in the West. This is in fact so vast a subject that we can do no more than undertake a cursory review of the topic. Those who want to go into more detail are referred to *The American Association of Oriental Medicine's Complete Guide to Chinese Herbal Medicine* by David Molony, *Spontaneous Healing* by Andrew Weil, and *Guide to Alternative Medicine* by Isadore Rosenfeld.

A major part of TCM is the practice of herbal medicine. The principles that govern TCM's understanding of the human body, namely, the interaction of yin and yang and the complex relationships between "wind," "cold," "heat," "damp," "dry," and "fire" are also used to categorize the substances prescribed to correct imbalances in the patient. The Chinese use a system of five rather than the four elements traditional in the West. These elements are earth, fire, water, metal, and wood. They are associated with the *zang* and *fu* organs (the heart is associated with fire, the kidney with water, for instance), with the divisions of the year, with emotions, and with specific properties of herbs, categorized often according to their flavors. In general, Chinese herbs have specific innate properties, some stimulating the yang and others the yin to balance their action and effects throughout the body.

The most famous ancient promoters of herbal medicine in China were the Divine Ploughman (the Emperor Sheng Yang) in 2800 B.C. and the Yellow Emperor (Huang Di) in 2687 B.C. The former was, in fact, the originator of the yin-yang concept. The latter authored *The Yellow Emperor's Classic of Internal Medicine*, upon which all TCM is based. Millennia of subsequent clinical observation and experiment have continued to employ the basic organizing categories of this ancient book.

Increased use of natural herbs is taking place in the United States, in the United Kingdom, in many European countries, throughout the East, and in the developing world. Wherever one travels in the West, not only in sophisticated cities but even in very small towns, one finds organic food stores with sections for herbal remedies. Many pharmacies today stock popular herbal products.

Americans spend several billions of dollars on herbal remedies each year. It is reckoned that eighty percent of the world's population relies on the use of herbal medicine. With the growing complexity, specialization, and cost of orthodox medical treatment, and the impersonal nature of conventional diagnosis and cure, herbal medicine is perceived to be a way one can take back control of one's own health.

With a little study, no more than reading pamphlets available in the local health food store, one can inform oneself about herbal remedies. In many stores the salespeople themselves are quite ready to give the customer some limited advice. In our opinion, some people who work in health food stores may be sources of valid information, but many are not. Members of the public are advised to consult their physician before taking any herbal products and only to purchase them from licensed and reputable vendors, upon the advice of their physician. Products that given singly may have no untoward effects may, when given in combination with another product, have an adverse effect, which may be serious in some instances.

In regard to Chinese herbs, one should be aware that in China the production of herbal drugs is uncontrolled, and that there is no monitoring system in the U.S. to insure the purity or safety of the herbs or the accuracy of their indicated strengths, whether manufactured in China or in the U.S. In the United Kingdom, France, Germany, and many other parts of Europe, there are such monitoring systems in place.

I hope that the following list of herbal remedies will be useful to the reader. This list combines Chinese and Western products and gives conditions that they may help to relieve.

*Aconite* to stimulate metabolism and tonify cardiac muscle
*Angelica:* type 1 relieves low back pain; type 2 is used for headaches and
    sore throats; type 3 regulates female reproductive organs
*Asparagus* for dry coughs
*Aspirin* from willow bark for fever and to relieve pain
*Atropine* from Belladonna, an antispasmodic
*Bamboo leaf* for urinary infections
*Camomile* tea for relaxation, insomnia, irritability, colic, and aid digestion
*Cardamom seed* for poor digestion
*Cinnamon bark* for chronic diarrhea
*Citrus peel* for indigestion and to increase metabolism

*Dianthus* for urinary infections, irregular menstruation, and constipation

*Digitalis* from the foxglove for tachycardia, atrial fibrillation, and congestive heart failure

*Dragon blood* to stop bleeding

*Echinacea* for protection against colds and to stimulate the immune system

*Ephedrine* from ephedra, an antispasmodic, but a potentially dangerous drug

*Evening primrose oil* contains fatty acids, is used in treating heart disease, is thought to be better than a placebo

*Fennel* to stimulate digestive organs

*Feverfew* for migraines

*Forsythia* for colds and fevers

*Gardenia fruit* for bladder infections, jaundice, ulcers, and irritability

*Garlic* to lower blood cholesterol and lower blood pressure

*Ginger root* to prevent nausea, headaches, vomiting, and colds

*Gingko seeds* for coughs, asthma, tuberculosis, and bladder infections; an antioxidant and free-radical destroyer, thought to increase blood flow and help in Reynaud's disease

*Ginseng root* to treat yang deficiencies, tonify qi, enhance the immune system, improve sex life, increase energy, stimulate and strengthen the immune system; thus possibly can prevent cancer

*Green teas* for asthma and to prevent cancer (four to six cups a day)

*Licorice* to harmonize other herbs, as an anti-inflammatory and anti-cancer drug (use with great care, as it can induce hypertension)

*Morphine* from the poppy to relieve pain

*Saw palmetto* contains fatty acid extracts, helps build body weight during convalescence, increases libido, sexuality, and sperm formation; it is used to reduce prostatic enlargement (this takes two to three months of administration)

*Senna pods* for constipation

*Tonics* such garlic, ginger, green tea, ginseng, and maitake mushrooms are all thought to increase the efficiency of the healing system

*Valerian* as a sedative and mood improver

The following formulas for combinations of two or more herbs are given to correct imbalances that result in common ailments.

*For alcoholism*, ginseng and atractylodes
*For allergies*, ma huang, xanthine, and magnolia
*For arthritis*, pueraria combination, clematis, and corydalis
*For asthma*, ma huang, ginseng, and astragalus
*For back pain*, rehmannia and gentian
*For colds/flu*, lonicera and forsythia
*For constipation*, apricot seed and linum
*For diarrhea*, ayastache and gentian
*For ear infections*, rhododendron and gentian
*For gallstones*, rhubarb and sartellaria
*For hypertension*, ginseng and longan
*For the immune system*, ginseng and rehmannia 6
*For indigestion*, citrus and pirsellia
*For insomnia*, ginseng and zirzyphna
*For menopause*, buplurum and dragon bone
*For urinary infections*, dianthus and corydalis
*For yeast infections*, tang gui and ginseng 8

While all health professionals should keep an open mind when considering ideas that are new to them, the purchaser or patient is advised to consult a reputable physician or therapist before using any herbal product. This is particularly so when dealing with combinations of two or more products.

# – 10 –

# Naturopathy

NATUROPATHY IS A FORM of holistic, alternative medicine, originally formulated by nineteenth-century European physicians and emphasizing "natural" processes of healing, that is, healing without drugs or surgery. Naturopathic physicians hold that there is a healing force in nature (*vis medicatrix naturae*) which allows the body to heal itself. This ability can be enhanced with the support of diet, herbs, and supplements such as vitamins, and through the implementation of exercise, hydrotherapy, massage, relaxation, and counseling.

Naturopathy came to North America in 1905 when Benedict Lust, a German immigrant, established the first school of naturopathic medicine in New York State. He himself was inspired by the work of German therapists such as Father Sebastian Kneipp, one of the enthusiastic supporters of naturopathy on the European continent.

The roots of the naturopathic attitude toward healing lie deep in the medical tradition and take us back to both ancient Chinese medicine and to the work of Hippocrates and his coworkers in ancient Greece. The development of naturopathy in modern Europe owes something to the popularity of fashionable health spas over the last few hundred years—places like Aix-les Bains in France or Bath and Droitwich in Britain, where those who could afford it went to "take the waters," unpleasant to the taste though they were. Those seeking more robust health would spend weeks at such places, which were usually established in agreeable rural settings and often provided the opportunity to consult not only with physicians but with other persons with reputations as healers, and not only about their physical maladies but about the stress of life and emotional problems.

In connection with these spas, it was thought that certain natural environments were particularly conducive to returning the ill to health. The clean, open air and sunshine of the Swiss mountains, for instance, were considered beneficial for treating tuberculosis. Bathing in the sea was also believed to have curative effects. This latter concept led to the founding of sea bathing hospitals at Margate in England and at Berck Plage in France, which are flourishing orthopedic hospitals today. Some years ago one of us visited the hospital at Berck Plage, now a place for long-term treatment of orthopedic conditions, such as scoliosis in children. The claims of the spas to cure disease were exaggerated, but the belief in a healthy environment does indeed have considerable influence on maintaining health.

The history of public interest in the naturopathic attitude toward healing over the past hundred years illustrates well the notion that there is a pendulum-like alternation in human affairs. During the early decades of the twentieth century, the general public embraced naturopathy. Popularity allowed it to increase its scope and its number of practitioners and to open some twenty schools, which offered programs of training in its practices and point of view. Between 1925 and 1950 the discipline became recognized in four Canadian provinces. But after the second World War, the discovery of miracle drugs such as penicillin and streptomycin and the rapid development of new surgical techniques led to the general confidence that conventional medical science would soon be able understand and treat virtually all disease. Interest in naturopathic medicine, with its emphasis on healing without such external remedies as drugs and surgery, waned.

In the past thirty years the pendulum has swung once again, as it has become clear that, in spite of many victories, medical science does not have all the answers regarding health and healing. We are all too keenly aware that surgery and pharmaceuticals create health problems of their own, are often far from cost-effective, and in any case do not represent anything like a complete picture of our healing capabilities. Accordingly, both in the U.S. and in Canada there has been a marked renewal of interest in the power of natural medicine.

The principles on which naturopathic medicine is based are as follows:

1. There is a healing power in nature, inherent in all living organisms, which establishes, maintains, and restores health.
2. The causes of illness must be identified and removed before healing can occur.
3. The physician should use methods that offer the least risk of harmful effects. This in fact confirms the Hippocratic injunction: "Do no harm."
4. The physician should not seek the suppression of symptoms.
5. The physician is truly a doctor, the word doctor in Latin meaning "teacher." The physician's job is to educate the patient to take responsibility for his or her health.
6. The physician should treat the whole person, taking into account the physical, mental, emotional, social, and environmental aspects of each medical problem.
7. Prime emphasis should be placed on prevention. This involves a concern for the environment. A person cannot be healthy in an unhealthy environment.
8. Naturopathic practice must remain open to the full variety of effective healing modalities.
9. In applying the above principles, the individual condition and needs of each patient must be recognized.

Beyond this point naturopaths generally express the point of view that an inner conviction of spiritual values can be very important in the treatment of cancer and other chronic illnesses. Sir John Polkinghorne, scientist and theologian, has said that the widespread religious unbelief in the contemporary Western world is a limited phenomenon, both historically and geographically. Study of the work of the members of this profession reminds us that science and religion are in fact cousins, that God created the world through evolution, that intuition is as important as logic, that each one of us has a right side of the brain as well as a left, and that those of us in conventional medicine need to know a good deal more than we do about the beliefs and work of others in alternative and complementary medicine.

Naturopathic physicians are usually general practitioners, working either singly, in pairs, or with other health practitioners, such as M.D.s, D.C.s and D.O.s, in multidisciplinary clinics. Some, of course, also teach at the naturopathic colleges. Though naturopathic medicine emphasizes the ability of the individual to heal him or herself, it is not dogmatically opposed to the application of medical intervention as practiced by other disciplines, when appropriate. Naturopathy has already forged links with conventional medicine, with Chinese medicine and acupuncture, with chiropractic, osteopathy, and homeopathy. As we will see, familiarity with these disciplines is part of the naturopathic physician's formal training.

Many naturopathic doctors are particularly interested in complementary practices for the treatment of cancer. They are first of all very concerned with the role of diet and nutrition in a comprehensive cancer healing program. The cancer patient's diet should consist of whole foods that have a high fiber content and are low in sugar. It should avoid red meat but include some fish. The diet should be high in fresh, organically grown vegetables, fresh fruit, and fruit juices. Naturopaths also stress the very great value of vitamins in adequate doses; in particular, mineral complements with selenium, zinc, N-acetyl cysteine, and co-enzyme Q10 are highly desirable. The consumption of green teas, flavonoids, and specially grown mushrooms are also advocated.

Naturopaths concerned with the treatment of cancer place strong emphasis on the patient's emotional and mental attitude and on his or her belief system. They consider that the treatment of the mind of the patient is at least as important as the others aspects of treatment. They believe, and we think rightly, that a confident, optimistic attitude is particularly important in maintaining a healthy immune system which, as we have seen, is the main defense the body has against malignant cells.

Maintaining a confident attitude after one has been diagnosed with a life-threatening disease like cancer is not easy, and many naturopathic physicians have recourse to biofeedback, guided imagery, meditation, and progressive relaxation therapy to this end. Another way to maintain a confident attitude is for the patient to take an active role in his or her own healing process. Naturopaths therefore take time to educate the patient in the nature of his or her disease and how they can work to deal with it. A naturopath we know has this as a working motto, "I am the navigator; the patient is the pilot."

Taking charge of the healing process requires making major lifestyle changes—changes in diet, as we have seen, in exercise, in personal priorities, in one's beliefs, and in one's relationships. Such a major overhaul of the way one lives may sometimes seem to throw one's entire existence into disarray. But we know from chaos theory that the appearance of disorder may be an opportunity for a step toward a deeper state of order. The naturopathic physician helps patients to keep their bearings through this period of disorientation, and acts on the principle that a small change at the start can lead to a big change at the end.

At the time of this writing there are two naturopathic colleges in North America, one in Portland, Oregon, and one in Bothel, a few miles north of Seattle, Washington. There are two more that expect accreditation and recognition in the near future, in Toronto and in Tempe, Arizona.

The National College in Portland Oregon, which offers a four-year program, is fully accredited for granting the degree of N.D. (Doctor of Naturopathy). To qualify for admission candidates must have a B.S. degree or the equivalent. This college also offers training toward the degree of Master of Science in Oriental Medicine (M.S.O.M.).

Bastyr University in Bothel, a few miles north of Seattle on the eastern shore of Lake Washington, is also fully accredited. The admission requirements are the same as for the National College. The course for the N.D. degree is of four years duration. The university also offers degrees of

Master of Science in Nutrition, in Acupuncture, and in Oriental Medicine; a Bachelor of Science in Applied Behavioral Sciences; and a Master of Arts in Applied Behavioral Sciences.

The Canadian College of Naturopathic Medicine in Toronto expects to gain full accreditation shortly. The admission requirements and the length of the course towards the N.D. degree are the same as in the two institutions mentioned above. Southwest College of Naturopathic Medicine in Tempe, Arizona, has been open since 1992 and is on the path to full accreditation.

The curricula for the N.D. degree in the four existing colleges are almost identical. In the first year there are eighteen courses, in the second year fifteen, in the third year seventeen, and in the fourth year seven, with extra clinical work. In the first year many of the courses are similar to those in an M.D. program in any medical school, but there are also courses in botanical medicine, homeopathy, naturopathic history and philosophy, oriental medicine, and hydrotherapy. During the second year many of the courses are also the same as in conventional medicine but with additional courses in homeopathy, nutrition, oriental medicine and acupuncture, oriental medicine and naturopathic manipulation.

For the third year a number of courses are virtually the same as in a conventional medical school, with additional courses again in homeopathy, orthopedics, manipulation, and oriental medicine, and the remainder in naturopathic manipulation, obstetrics, pediatrics, emergency care, counseling, and ethics. In the final year there are seven courses in clinical work, practice management, ethics, communicating skills, treatment modalities, integrated clinical studies, and minor surgery. The uninitiated may well wonder how students are able to master so many diverse subjects.

Study of the present setup in naturopathy and of the curricula for the N.D. degree has involved us in some hard work, which has been rewarding in that it has opened our eyes to what to us has been a new development. As we look to the future with this new information in mind, there are several conclusions that seem to be of great importance: Here are people who mean business. Naturopathic physicians are serious medical practitioners with a clear vision of how to develop their approach to healing. What they propose does not conflict with the things conventional medicine does well. In their emphasis on prevention, simple natural methods, teaching patients to care for themselves, the importance of the environment, getting alongside the patient, and considering the value of other complementary and alternative forms of medicine, naturopathy has much to teach those of us who are trained in conventional medicine alone. In several respects they are ahead of us.

As practitioners of an orthodox variety of medicine, we are impressed for the most part with what we've been able to learn about naturopathy. We do have one question, however. Naturopathic physicians, in common with practitioners of complementary disciplines, are very concerned about the buildup of toxic substances in the body and consequently recommend methods of detoxification. One frequently applied technique is "colonic lavage"—a special kind of enema using a large quantity of water, administered with the aim of detoxifying the patient. As far as we can see, however, naturopathic physicians neither identify the toxic substances nor specify why colonic lavage is given such a prominent place in their repertoire of practices. Is this really necessary, in view of the fact that the colon sheds its lining almost daily? Large doses of vitamin C would appear to do the job quite thoroughly. Our objection is not a radical one, but we would ourselves hesitate to undergo colonic lavage without a very convincing reason for its use.

We find it of great interest that naturopathy has culled concepts from disciplines as diverse as acupuncture, chiropractic, conventional, homeopathic, oriental, and osteopathic medicine. It is encouraging to discover that therapists from these very different areas are learning to work in cooperation and are apparently enjoying the process.

There is a giant clam that lives in the depths of the sea, where light is very poor. Living with it, between the sides of the shell, is one of the green algae. Tiny mirrors on the clam's shell focus the light that the alga needs for photosynthesis, and the clam too benefits from this—a thoroughly good and profitable kind of cooperation. The boxer crab lives under rock at a depth of four meters in the Indian and Pacific Oceans and the Red Sea. This crab forms a home for a pair of stinging sea anemones in its claws, which it uses to defend itself by immobilizing its prey—a form of cooperation that is not so benign. The members of our diverse disciplines need to be quite certain that our cooperation is entirely for the benefit of our patients, ourselves and our communities rather than to advance our own particular interests to the detriment of others.

We dare to suggest that it might be of benefit to seek a new name for the discipline of naturopathy. A new name would suggest a new way of thinking, commensurate with the new outlook that is the hallmark of this discipline.

# – 11 –

# Aromatherapy

A N INTUITIVE AWARENESS of the connection between aromas and health has been part of folk medicine for millennia. The aroma of hot chicken soup (as Maimonides taught and as millions of Jewish mothers have practiced) probably has a more beneficial affect on the nasal mucosa than the medically recommended inhalation of steam from hot water. The most delightful aroma of the day is that of coffee beans being ground for breakfast coffee. This is almost more pleasing than the first sip of the fresh-brewed drink itself! How can there be the slightest doubt of the value of aromatherapy?

Aromatherapy is the art and science of using essential oils to help balance and heal our bodies, minds, and spirits. Essential oils are concentrated extracts of the roots, leaves, flowers, fruit, and bark of plants and trees. Neither we nor others who are interested in aromatherapy believe that it is a primary modality in the treatment of serious disease. But we do believe that certain aromatic, essential oils can relieve stress, can improve the patient's mood, and can be an important indirect factor in the healing process.

The effect upon mood is not merely psychological. Our sensory receptors for smell are hairlike processes that are situated in the upper nasal passages. These receptors, when activated, send messages to the limbic system in the brain—the seat of emotion, memory, and sexual arousal. The limbic system is connected to the physical responses associated with these psychological phenomena. Thus the response to an aroma can affect blood pressure, heart rate, breathing, and perhaps the immune system. We do not, however, agree with those who advocate the use of essential oils as antibiotics.

One day in the 1920s a French chemist, Rene-Maurice Gattefosse, burned his hand badly and immediately plunged it into a jar of lavender oil. The pain subsided almost at once, and the burn healed very quickly, without leaving a scar. The chemist's interest was piqued. After some experimentation he found that other oils had a similar potential for healing, not only burn wounds but some skin disorders as well. Another French doctor, Jean Valnet, independently used essential oils for conditions not directly related to the skin, such as insomnia, anxiety, and stress. The essential oils, of course, gave off noticeable aromas, and the idea arose that the healing properties of the oils might also belong to the aromas as such. Toward the end of nineteenth century Valnet published a book in French, which was translated into English as *The Practice of Aromatherapy* and had some influence in generating interest in the use of aromatic oils for healing.

Today, there are about forty aromatic essential oils that aromatherapists apply in hot baths or through the skin during massage. A few drops of an aromatic oil added to a hot bath do indeed have a very soothing effect. And oils like chamomile and lavender, diluted in a base such as almond oil, can be an effective addition when applied to the skin before massage. We all know that massage is very effective in the treatment of bruises, sprains, strains, and allied conditions. It is even more so if a few drops of the appropriate oil are rubbed on the skin at the outset.

There are many examples of the specific healing effects of the application of aromatic oils. Arnica helps the relief of athletic injuries, olive oil warms and soothes, and eucalyptus oil is a good adjuvant for inhaling in steam for infections of the nose, throat, and bronchi. It is said that the aroma of vanilla helps to lessen the claustrophobia experienced during

MRI, when the patient is restrained in a very confined space. Some practitioners have found that oil of lavender is useful for patients in intensive care after a heart attack. It is suggested that the aroma coming from lavender oil or licorice may have a role in the treatment of impotence by influencing the dilatation of the blood vessels to the penis.

From these examples it is obvious that the effectiveness of aromatherapy goes beyond the merely subjective sensations of pleasure that aromas may arouse. Aromatherapists are sensitive that their science not be confused with the multi-million dollar cosmetics industry that, like aromatherapy itself, has emanated mainly from France.

This is not to say that subjective olfactory experiences are not in themselves health factors. The medicinal odors in doctors' offices contribute to an atmosphere of anxiety for many patients, which can be relieved by the presence of more pleasant scents. Orthodox physicians could benefit from giving more attention to the medical environment and attempt to make their clinics and offices more attractive and less overwhelming to their patients.

Aromatherapy is certainly not a powerful or aggressive agent in fighting disease. But, after all, the vast majority of problems that make us feel ill are very minor ones and do not necessarily require powerful and aggressive remedies. It's only sensible that the doctor or other therapist do everything possible to relieve the patient's discomfort and give him or her a feeling of well-being.

It is clear that the study required to become an aromatherapist is much less demanding than, for example, that required to become a chiropractor, but some training is necessary and readily available. It is usually presented as part of the training to become licensed in massage. Courses usually involve four hours per week for sixteen weeks, independent of the requirements for qualification in massage therapy. A varying number of practical case studies are required after the theoretical course is completed. When the course and case studies are successfully completed, the therapist can practice either as a self-employed aromatherapist or for an institution. Aromatherapy courses in some countries are internationally recognized, but in other cases a further qualification is required.

As we have seen, there may be some ailments for which aromatherapy can be applied as a primary remedy. In such cases, it is up to the patient to decide whether to go with aromatherapy or conventional care, and we can properly think of aromatherapy as "alternative medicine." But for the most part, aromatherapy is useful as an enhancement conducive to healing and should be thought of as complementary, not alternative, medicine.

It is perhaps best to think of aromatherapy as providing one of the "little nudges" toward health—small initial interventions that, if applied at the right moment can produce far-reaching final results. To see it this way helps us to accept many therapeutic measures that in truth we cannot measure!

# — 12 —

# Miscellaneous Disciplines

THE MAIN PURPOSE of this book is not to describe every possible alternate or complementary kind of medicine, but rather to enable the reader the better to understand how conventional and complementary disciplines relate to and interact with one another. That one or another kind of complementary discipline is not mentioned does not mean it is not important. In this chapter we'll make brief mention of a number of other complementary and alternative disciplines.

## Ayurveda

Eastern medical philosophies, with their emphasis on hope and humanity, are becoming increasingly popular, in spite of their not being regarded as scientific. One such approach to medicine originating in India that is becoming better and better known in the west is ayurvedic medicine. In India itself approximately eighty percent of the population has its medical care from ayurvedic practitioners. The word *ayurveda* means "knowledge of life." In the ayurvedic philosophy of medicine, every person is considered to be a combination of mind, body, senses, and soul.

The soul is understood to be composed of a vital energy called *prana* in Sanskrit. Prana is roughly the equivalent of the Chinese *qi*. As in most philosophies originating in India, ayurvedic medicine recognizes the principle of reincarnation or rebirth. When we die, the soul is believed to be reborn in the body of what is essentially another person. Each person is a combination of three different forces, which combine to determine one's characteristics, which in turn determine how one should conduct one's life. Since these forces combine differently in each individual, the prescription for a healthy life has to be individually tailored.

Ayurvedic doctors are trained in diet, cooking, and meditation, and familiarize themselves with the qualities of a large number of herbs. Medical significance is attached to a patient's environment and to what clothes he or she wears. Lack of balance in one's life is believed to be the prime cause of illness, and, in general, more emphasis is placed on prevention than on treatment. Drinking several glasses of hot water each day is recommended for everyone, and though culinary requirements for each person are a very individual matter, eating the correct foods is considered to be of great importance for all.

Ayurvedic treatment itself emphasizes detoxification, which may be performed by inducing vomiting, by purging, and by applying enemas, steam baths, or healing herbs. Massage is often applied to specific parts of the body and specific breathing and yoga exercises are often assigned. There seems to be no scientific proof of the effectiveness of ayurvedic medicine, though the newly appointed Office of Alternative Medicine of the N.I.H. is now supporting research into its principles.

The emphasis ayurvedic medicine places on lifestyle and the avoidance of stress is something that it shares with many medical disciplines, whether traditional, orthodox, or complementary, though we must say that some of its remedies—the use of enemas of ground up peacock testicles to treat impotence comes to mind—seem quite nonsensical. We can certainly agree with Eastern people who believe in ayurvedic medicine that a healthy lifestyle that includes time for meditation and relaxation is of great value. In the West increasing numbers of M.D.s, chiropractors, naturopaths, nurses, and osteopaths are familiarizing themselves with ayurvedic methods.

# Chelation

Chelation is a very controversial technique for treating patients with constriction of the arteries of the heart or legs that avoids the need for costly and dangerous angioplasty or bypass surgery. Chelation (from the Greek *chele*, meaning "claw") is based on observations that when a certain amino-acid complex (ethylene diamine tetra acetic acid or EDTA) comes into contact with positively charged metals such as lead or iron, it "grabs" them like a claw. Chelation is thus the approved way of treating lead and other forms of heavy metal poisoning. When EDTA is injected into the bloodstream of a person suffering from metal poisoning, it combines with the metal and removes it so it can be easily excreted by the kidneys.

Some doctors, thinking that EDTA might be helpful for patients with constricted arteries due to calcification in atherosclerotic plaques, conducted experiments on rabbits in whom atherosclerosis had been induced by high-cholesterol diets. They found that with this treatment the plaques melted away. It was suggested that EDTA might be equally effective in treating narrowed arteries in human patients.

Thousands of doctors now chelate over 500,000 people each year, but authorities in the F.D.A., N.I.H., and A.M.A. are of the opinion that the benefits of chelation are at best unproved, and that the procedure is ineffective and in fact dangerous. The decrease in size of the plaques in rabbits has not been demonstrated in human patients, and it is argued that the substances that narrow the artery are cholesterol and scar tissue, which contain very little calcium.

In double-blind studies using controls and patients treated by chelation, there was no difference in the blood flow through the arteries experienced by the two groups, though both reported improvement in symptoms. It has been suggested that other measures such as exercise, stopping smoking, and loss of weight, which were documented in both groups at the same time as the chelation, were responsible for the improvement and not the chelation itself. Many patients, however, do report considerable benefit from chelation, and it would be foolish to condemn the procedure out of hand. Further controlled studies are called for.

# Magnetic Therapy

The study of physics tells us that there are four forces that operate in the universe: gravity, electromagnetism, and the "large" and the "weak" nuclear forces. The strong and weak forces are operative within the nucleus of the atom and within the elementary particles themselves and do not affect us directly, except insofar as we are exposed to atomic radiation. Electromagnetism and gravity permeate every aspect of our existence. In the nineteenth century physicists demonstrated that the force of attraction and repulsion that make magnets work and the force of electricity are two aspects of the same thing. That is why today we speak of "electromagnetism" or the "electromagnetic force." Electromagnetism keeps us from falling apart: it is responsible for the bonds that hold atoms together in all chemical molecules.

Gravity is a force of attraction between all bodies that have mass or material substance. It affects us constantly while we are on the earth, as well as being the primary reason that star systems and galaxies hold together and have the forms they do. The delicate balance between gravity and electromagnetism makes stars burn uniformly and last for very long periods.

Scientists tell us that our bodies are surrounded by an electromagnetic field. There is no doubt that electromagnetism affects us to a considerable degree, just as gravity does. Our body's energy processes generate their own magnetic fields, which can be detected and measured. The human brain emits electrical currents of two cycles per second while we're asleep and up to twenty cycles per second while we're awake. Magnetic resonance imaging (MRI) works because it interprets our bodies' magnetic energy.

The pervasiveness of electromagnetic energy has given rise to both fears and hopes. Some people fear that exposure to magnetic energy can make us ill, and there is some evidence that living near an electric power station, for instance, may be associated with an increased risk of leukemia. There is no hard evidence that electromagnetic energy from microwaves, electric razors, or fluorescent lighting has harmful effects.

On the other hand, some writers believe that magnetic field therapy can be used to treat disorders ranging from stress to cancer. There is indeed good evidence that this kind of therapy can be used to enhance the healing of fractures. We have talked to patients with painful joints, for example from arthritis affecting the ankle, who have experienced very marked relief from wearing a magnet over the painful area. For this kind of use, magnets are readily available that can be strapped around the affected part of the body. Some people believe that they sleep better and feel better with a magnet under the pillow.

There is an increasing amount of interest in the therapeutic value of electromagnetism, especially in the area of pain control. We would not attempt to discourage the use of this kind of therapy. It is a useful "little nudge" for the clinician dealing with a patient who has not responded to other measures.

Dr. Richard Gerber, who practices internal medicine at Michigan State, has written at some length on an allied topic in his book *Vibrational Medicine*. For the present writers this is a fascinating topic, though Dr. Gerber's book is difficult to absorb. *Publishers Weekly* writes that it "is at the cutting edge of the whole health movement." The well-known medical author Dr. Larry Dossey writes that "the combination of ancient wisdom and new science is the definitive introduction to health care for modern times." He goes on to write that Dr. Gerber's encyclopedic treatment of subtle energy fields, acupuncture, Bach flower remedies, crystals, radionics, chakras, meditation, and homeopathy has achieved widespread acceptance by many institutions across the United States.

Dr. Dossey thinks further that Dr. Gerber has provided a valuable step in thinking beyond biomechanics and into the domain of mind and spirit and shows how this domain will become a crucial factor in the medicine of the future. Dr. Norman Shealy of the American Holistic Medical Association writes that "the book covers extremely well the transition from science to metaphysics and will serve as a useful guide to those ready to begin the path toward energy and consciousness. This is a good example for those individuals who are beginning to open their consciousness."

The practitioner of present-day conventional medicine will, like ourselves, find the concepts discussed in this book hard to grasp. That doesn't mean that they are not important. It is good that we be prepared to consider things outside our present ken. This reminds us of a very important thing, so often forgotten: that no one of us has the time or energy or ability to become conversant in every discipline in health care. We can include three or four different fields of study and practice in our practical armamentarium and remain wise and humble enough to concede the potential value of matters we don't yet comprehend.

# Mind-Body Therapy

Quantum theory teaches us that the mind and the body are a unity. The mind can affect the body, and the body can affect the mind. A fright can produce an increase in the heart rate and in the blood pressure. Mental stress produces definite physical effects and probably depresses the immune system. The immune system, of course, helps to prevent infections and to eliminate cancerous cells. The chemical substances that are part of this system have been identified. At the same time we are beginning to understand how specific chemical substances (neuropeptides) may be associated with specific emotional states.

As a result of these developments, a new discipline, psychoneuroimmunology, has emerged over the past decade which enhances our knowledge of the relationship between mind and body. It studies how the mind, the nervous system, and the hormones are able to enhance the activity of the immune system. Three approaches to therapy that make use of these new ways of understanding the relation between mind and body are biofeedback, guided imagery, and meditation. While biofeedback is a new technique that developed with the use of technological instruments for measuring psychophysical states, guided imagery and meditation are traditional practices whose potentialities for healing have only been recognized by the orthodox, scientific medical community since the advent of psychoneuroimmunology.

*Biofeedback* is employed by therapists in both conventional and complementary medicine. Many studies have been carried out on this subject. There are differences of opinion as to how it works, but there is no doubt that it is a useful procedure in many cases.

Normally, the autonomic nervous system, which controls such essential functions in the body as heart rate, blood pressure, respiration, and the functioning of the intestinal tract is not under conscious control. With biofeedback techniques some measure of voluntary access to these functions is apparently achievable. The technique works as follows. Electrodes (electronic sensing devices) are attached to the skin to receive information about the heart, the pulse, blood pressure, muscle tension, and skin temperature. The electrodes are connected to a recording instrument to measure the intensity of the process being monitored. The patient listens to the tone or watches the display on the instrument's meter or screen and concentrates his or her attention, in an attempt to influence the process under study, for example the blood pressure.

How control is gained is not known, but the process of getting "feedback" from one's own body through seeing its functioning monitored in this way seems to allow many people to find an intuitive means to make the readings change in the desired direction. This might occur by the patient's visualizing scenes or objects that ordinarily affect how he or she feels, while at the same time "willing" to decrease the pulse rate or the blood pressure, to make a headache go away, or to reduce stress, as the case may be. It usually takes eight or nine sessions to become conversant with the process.

Biofeedback is not always successful, but is often effective in the treatment of high blood pressure, tension headaches, and Reynaud's syndrome. (The latter is a disturbance of the sympathetic nervous system which results in contraction of the small arteries to the hands and feet, with pain and blanching of the affected part. The patient is very sensitive to cold and has repeated attacks of the syndrome, which may lead to necrosis of the fingers and toes. It is always troublesome and may be serious.)

*Guided imagery* is an approach that is useful in reducing anxiety, in improving the patient's mood, and in easing pain, especially from cancer.

The patient forms a mental image and attempts to focus the subconscious on making it seem real. In fact, ordinary daydreaming and fantasizing generate images and affect us by the same process as guided imagery. For instance, an exciting thought can increase the pulse rate, or a sexual fantasy can produce an erection. The only difference is that in daydreams the image-making process is unguided and spontaneous and is just as likely to be motivated by a negative or fearful intention as by a positive and healing one. In guided imagery, this process is enlisted to generate positive results or to stimulate healing processes appropriate to the patient's illness.

Patients with cancer, for instance, can try to make mental pictures of the cells and chemicals of the immune system attacking and killing the cancer cells. It is often helpful to imagine the cells of the immune system as soldiers in an army that is attacking and killing the forces of the enemy. This process may in some cases actually result in reduction in the extent of the cancer, but in any case help is gained in improving the outlook and general well-being of the patient by marshaling his or her creative participation and thus overcoming a sense of helplessness. This indirectly supports the body's ability to fight the disease. In other conditions focusing on the painful area and imagining reduction of the symptoms can be very helpful. Making an image of a stroll in pleasant country on a fresh but warm summer day can have a very relaxing effect. Concentrating on breathing slowly and deeply calms the anxious person.

***Meditation and relaxation.*** Eastern religions have over the centuries developed many methods of focusing the mind and entering into states of meditation. Meditation both deepens and is deepened by relaxation. The process of relaxation can be pursued by individuals on their own or with groups of people. The Zen sitting of Buddhism, the yoga exercises recommended by ayurvedic medicine, Transcendental Meditation as taught in the West since the 1960s, and the "relaxation response" advocated by Herbert Benson of Harvard are all examples of meditation. It has been demonstrated that the last of these can moderate the production of the stress hormone cortisol, can allay anxiety, can help in the reduction of chronic pain, can lower blood cholesterol, can help in reducing substance abuse, and perhaps in some instances can prolong life.

One way of practicing meditation is to set aside two periods of time each day of thirty to forty minutes. The meditator sits in a comfortable chair with feet on the floor and breathes in and out slowly and deeply for a minute. The individual chooses a *mantra*—a short word, phrase, or syllable. It can be just about anything. The word "one" is recommended by Dr. Benson. The mantra is repeated inwardly, silently, and slowly, as one breathes in and out. The person becomes relaxed and unaware of the surroundings. When stray thoughts occur, the individual accepts them and returns to the mantra. The patient feels progressively better and more and more aware of the "inner self." The symptoms of stress fade away.

The effects of meditation can also be produced through prayer, through artistic activity such as painting or playing music, and by therapeutic touch. (Therapeutic touch, an art quite easy to acquire, works much like meditation and is an efficient way of relieving pain.) I (WHK-W) like to paint with acrylics, and I become relaxed and completely absorbed in what I'm doing. I like to do it with a mug of beer at hand. Sometimes I find I'm about to put my brush into the beer and drink the water I use to mix the paints! (The reader can draw his or her own conclusions about the writer!) On one occasion I let a bee sting me on the nose because I was too absorbed to interrupt my painting—but I didn't feel much pain and went on with my masterpiece!

# Reflexology

Reflexology, used in China five thousand years ago and introduced to the West early in the twentieth century by Dr. William Fitzgerald, is a widely recognized form of complementary medicine. Fitzgerald was an ear, nose, and throat surgeon who noticed that when pressure is applied to the palms of the hands or the soles of the feet just before surgery, the postoperative pain is greatly reduced.

Eunice Ingham, a massage therapist and physical medicine practitioner, expanded upon Fitzgerald's work. She thought that the pressure did not only reduce pain but improved many conditions such as diarrhea, constipation, migraine, asthma, allergic reactions, skin lesions, and tension. There are complicated theories as to how reflexology works which, to our minds, are not very convincing, and we need not trouble ourselves with them now. A treatment session lasts about forty-five minutes, the patient sitting with the legs raised. It is usual to have six weekly sessions for four to six weeks.

Practitioners of the art recommend that it should not be applied when the feet or hands are infected, when the patient has a fever, and in cases of phlebitis. It should be reserved for people with a condition that is not serious, such as migraine or an irritable bowel, when other therapies have not worked satisfactorily. Many patients enjoy reflexology and find it relaxing, leaving them with a feeling of well being which, as we have said many times, in itself is conducive to proper functioning of the immune system and hence good health.

# OTHER CONSIDERATIONS

# – 13 –

# The Immune System

IT IS IMPORTANT for all medical practitioners to understand something about our mysterious immune system and how it works. The cells of this system are scattered throughout the body, so medical practitioners of every specialty must make it part of their concern. Traditional allopathic medicine held that all illness enters the body from outside, and that the physician's main job is to attack the invader and demolish it.

Increasingly today, however, we understand that an equally important task is to prevent illness by promoting health. The body itself has a system for doing this: the immune system, in technical language, the reticulo-endothelial system. Since many forms of alternative and complementary medicine emphasize prevention over treatment, the increased understanding of the importance of the immune system is one of the main reasons for increased openness by physicians and the general public to unconventional modalities of medical practice.

It is amazing and at the same time encouraging to know that each one of us has his or her own doctor right inside us, working to keep us healthy, advising us about the ways of achieving this, keeping a lookout for any sign of trouble, and cracking down on anything within us, dead or living, that is reducing our well-being or working to make us ill. This is the essential function of the immune system.

Concretely, the immune system's role is to eliminate potentially harmful substances from the body. These include harmful bacteria, viruses, malignant cells, and the body's own dead cells. There are thousands of different kinds of bacteria on the skin and in the cavities of our bodies, the great majority of them harmless, many of them actually essential for our well-being. Even the harmful forms are, for the most part, innocuous and only cause damage under certain conditions.

At the same time, at every moment of our lives thousands of the cells of one organ or another in the ordinary course of their reproduction are spontaneously undergoing mutations and producing aberrant, premalignant cells which, if not eliminated, will give rise to cancer. Also, normal cells throughout the body are themselves continually coming to the end of their lives. They too have to be eliminated. It is the job of the cells and chemicals of the immune system to deal with all these harmful, unwanted entities in the most summary way possible.

The cells that carry out the work of the immune system are the white blood cells, the leucocytes. These are produced in the bone marrow, where primitive stem cells differentiate into polymorphonuclear leucocytes, which have irregular "lobulated" nuclei; and lymphocytes, with small, round, central nuclei. The lobulated nuclei of the polymorphs enable them to take many shapes; that is why they are called polymorphs. When they are summoned to the site of an injury or bacterial infection by chemical, neural, or hormonal signals, they surround the bacteria, ingest them, and kill them. The polymorphs are called phagocytic cells, meaning cells that eat.

After the polymorphs have done their work, what remains is a mass of dead cells—dead polymorphs and bacteria. This mass is removed by large phagocytic cells called macrophages—large cells that eat whatever they can find! At this point very small bits of the bacteria they have killed are displayed on the surface of the macrophages, and these attract the lymphocytes. Now, the polymorphs and macrophages are nonspecific in their action—they attack any entity that they fail to recognize as part of their own organism. The lymphocytes, on the other hand, are designed to attack specifically identified foreign entities. Lymphocytes develop in the bone marrow into two types: B-cells and T-cells. B-cells act "at a distance" from the bacteria they are programmed to destroy. T-cells act on contact and destroy virus-infected tissue and malignant cells.

The B-cells lodge in the lymph nodes, spleen, tonsils, and gut and act at a distance through substances that they produce called antibodies. In dealing with a bacterial infection, the B-cell is transformed to become a plasma cell with a nucleus that has small dark areas like the numbers on a the face of a clock. The plasma cells generate the antibodies. Each antibody is designed to destroy a specific foreign substance called its antigen. It is as if each bacterium (each antigen) had a specific lock into which only a specific antibody key might fit.

The antibodies are shaped like the letter Y. When an antibody finds the bacterium that is its antigen, the upper two arms of the Y stick onto it, and the lower arm attaches to a protein complex called complement. The antibody-complement complex travels in the blood to search and destroy the bacterium. An invasion of a particular kind of bacterium is the stimulus for the plasma cell to multiply and make the appropriate keys for the lock.

When a particular infection has been eliminated by particular antibodies, the work of the immune system is not done. A certain number of the B-cells keyed to the specific infection remain in hiding and at the ready, set to come into action again should there be another invasion by the same organism. This lying in wait of the B-cells cloned during a previous infection is what it means to have become immune to that type of infection. The key for the second infection is already in existence, and thus the killing effect is quicker and greater.

The T-cells are produced from a transformation of lymphocytes that enter the thymus, a small organ behind the breastbone. Most of the T-cells function as destroyers and are known as "natural killer cells." The T-cells handle tissue that has been infected by viruses as well as malignant cells. A virus is much much smaller than a bacterium. It is little more than a strand of genetic material inside a protein coat. It is unable to reproduce on its own but must penetrate the cell wall of a cell in another organism and use this other cell's DNA to help it multiply. In this way one virus particle becomes thousands, the host cell dies, and the newly formed virus particles are scattered to neighboring cells, which they now enter and where they continue to multiply, causing further cell death.

Fortunately, in order to enter a cell, a virus has to leave its protein coat on the outside. The presence of the coat sends a signal to the passing T-cells. When one of the appropriate type bumps against the wall of the affected cell, it perforates it and kills both cell and virus particles. A single T-cell can only kill one virus-affected cell at a time, but each T-cell clones itself, just as the plasma cells do. The clones disperse through the blood and tissues where, encountering other infected cells, they kill the viruses within them. Most of the T-cells function in this way as killers, but there are certain T-cells that act as suppressors, telling the system when to take a rest; there are others that act as helpers, telling the system when to become more active.

Since the power of the immune system to kill harmful alien cells is strong, it is important that the immune system act only on cells that in fact are alien, or are no longer functioning properly as part of one's own body. To insure that the immune system will be able to distinguish between the body's own cells and invaders, every single cell of each one of us has an identification mark on its surface—a special arrangement of protein molecules that constitutes the biological uniqueness of the individual.

An individual organism's T-cells on patrol recognize the identification mark and know by this means all the cells that belong to its own body. When they come in contact with foreign material or a cell with a different identification mark, they go quickly into action. When a cell becomes malignant, it loses its identification mark. Thus malignant cells are no longer recognized by T-cells as belonging to its own organism. In some way a message is passed on to other circulating killer cells to rush to the area and attack and kill the cell that has become a traitor. Continually, in every part of the body, some cells are mutating, losing their normal function and becoming malignant. For this reason alone, without the constant vigilance and action of the immune system we wouldn't live very long.

So we come now to the crux of the matter. The primary task of preventive medicine is to maintain the health and strength of the immune system. How can this task be performed? It is useful at this point to review the "ripples" and "nudges" that we discussed in the first chapter—very small influences at the start of a process that can and often do result in big changes at the end of it—whether for good (nudges) or for ill (ripples). These could be aspects of life, personal habits, dispositions, or states of emotion that, in terms of our health, act as seemingly slight instigation of truly momentous effects.

Some examples of ripples are fear, anxiety, anger, uncertainty, boredom, and hurry. Some examples of nudges are listening, caring, laughter, explaining, encouraging, attention, and prayer.

Quite simply, the more we can do to reduce the strength of the ripples and to increase the effect of the nudges, the stronger our immune system will be. The immune system is extremely sensitive to these aspects of our existence. Each one of us can do a great deal to help ourselves by the use of the "positive thinking" advocated long ago by Dr. Norman Vincent Peale. Our family, friends, colleagues at work and at play, and the boss at the workplace can add by their attitude to the health and vigor of the immune system. All this sounds very simple, but it is of vital importance.

Another way to nudge the immune system to better functioning is by taking vitamin supplements in quantities beyond the minimum daily requirements. Linus Pauling, the distinguished chemist and Nobel Prize winner, has drawn our attention to the fact that the dose of vitamins required to prevent illnesses such as rickets, scurvy, and pernicious anemia is not sufficient to keep the immune system working at its best. Deficiency of the requisite vitamins results in impairment of the immune system. He believes that the vitamins required for the health of the immune system are vitamin A from b-carotene, vitamin B12, pantothenic acid, folic acid, and vitamin C. Opinions differ as to the best dosage.

Vitamin C has become increasingly well known as an immune-system booster. It assists immunity in the following ways: (1) It helps synthesize the molecules necessary for the functioning of immune system cells such as the molecules that comprise the antibodies. (2) It helps antibodies adhere to the antigens, preparing the former to destroy invaders when combined with a complement. (3) It aids in the synthesis of part of complement. (4) It is involved in the "complement cascade," a series of chemical reactions that lead to the destruction of harmful cells. (5) Its specific effects in relation to cancer are that it increases the motility of phagocytes, cells that ingest bacteria and other particles, and increases the activity of natural killer cells.

Gowland Hopkins, professor of biochemistry at Cambridge University in the early years of this century, was one of the pioneers, along with biochemist Szent-Gyorgyi from Budapest, in the discovery of the vitamins. As undergraduate students I (WHK-W) and one of my friends had digs at the end of Tennis Court Road. We had to cycle furiously down this road to the physiology lab each morning at 8:50, in order not to be late for the nine o'clock lecture. The biochemistry building was opposite our lab at the bottom of the road. The more ribald of our colleagues used to remind us that all the staff of the biochemistry lab were socialists, except for Professor Hopkins, who had too much sense, and Dr. Cole, one of the lecturers, whose wife wouldn't let him!

Years later I took my wife to visit Cambridge, and as we walked down Tennis Court Road I proudly pointed out to her the somewhat dilapidated red brick building where Hopkins discovered vitamins. Her response was, "I suppose that working in such appalling conditions he just had to discover vitamins, or the population of the city would have succumbed long ago." Over the years she has learned to value these vitamins for herself!

There are other substances besides the vitamins recommended by Dr. Pauling that, taken as food supplements, have been found to stimulate the action of the immune system: pancreatic enzymes to digest the coatings of mutant cells, gingko biloba, garlic, echinacea, essiac, ukrain (celendine), antioxidants to protect genetic material against free radicals, vitamin super B50, vitamin E, selenium, and zinc.

Beyond the use of food supplements, visualization or conscious imagery techniques can be helpful in acting as a little nudge to enhance the immune system. With these techniques, the individual relaxes and makes a picture in his or her mind of the cells and antibodies within, patroling the tissues of the body, recognizing cells that have become malignant or bacteria that are harmful, and then taking the required measures to destroy them . One can also make a picture of the tissues in the body as they are responding, to give the immune system greater strength and power. It is useful, when one is ill, to spend ten or fifteen minutes on this exercise daily.

Living a healthy lifestyle is also important for immune system hygiene. This involves taking adequate exercise, having enough sleep, having enjoyable hobbies, finding ways to relieve stress, maintaining a felicitous home life, and developing sensible eating habits. This last item means, basically, a low-fat, low-meat, low-sugar, low-dairy diet.

Besides being suppressed by the ripples mentioned on our list, the immune system can be suppressed through the body's exposure to toxins that accumulate through unhealthy habits or even our subjection to medical practices. Alcohol, nicotine, food additives, and excessive intake of fat, sugar, meat, and dairy products all suppress the immune system. But so do painkillers such as aspirin, acetaminiphen (Tylenol), ibuprofen (Advil), some antibiotics, and the major cancer therapies—chemotherapy, radiotherapy, and surgery.

Enhancement of our knowledge of the ways in which the immune system works is the subject of consideration in the new field of psychoneuroimmunology, which deals with the ways in which the emotions (nudges and ripples) connect with the immune system. These pathways along which the emotions affect our immune systems are partly hormonal (chemical) and partly neural (along the nerves).

We can now understand why, in general, physicians should seek the help of the immunologist, nutritionist, herbal therapist, naturopath, exercise therapist, and others for the purpose of boosting immunity for the prevention of disease, the maintenance of health, and the treatment of diseases such as infection and cancer. A healthy regard for the efficient functioning of the immune system is a very cogent reason for cooperation among those in different disciplines. We cannot manage without one another.

# – 14 –

# A Word About Cancer

NOTHING CAN SPEAK more strongly in favor of cooperation between the different branches of mainstream and complementary medicine than the prevention and treatment of cancer. In the first chapter we discussed how the nature of our universe itself suggests the wisdom of this cooperation. In the last chapter we discussed the role of the immune system in protecting the body against bacterial and viral invaders and against the cells of the body that have become malignant. It is fitting now to consider these very important matters further.

Every day of our lives some of our cells take a wrong turn and become malignant, potentially menacing the whole body. We've seen that this is inevitable, but that under normal conditions the cells and chemicals of the immune system are mobilized to detect and destroy these abnormal cells before they can do irreparable damage. A strong and healthy immune system is the best possible safeguard against the development of a malignant lesion. Under certain conditions, however, some of the abnormal cells escape detection and we have the onset of cancer.

Today when a person is diagnosed with cancer, he or she faces a series of daunting options: (1) medically approved, orthodox treatments that are painful, debilitating, and, though they do prolong life, are in the long run rarely completely successful; (2) an ever-expanding menu of alternative treatments that also promise to prolong life but with varying degrees of scientific validation; (3) no treatment at all, with almost certain death as the outcome.

How would we advise a member of our own family or a close friend if she told us that she had cancer? We'd find it very difficult to know what to say. A friend of ours in her eighties had bowel trouble. After adequate investigation she was diagnosed with cancer of the colon that had spread to the liver. She was told that, without treatment, she had only a short time to live. She went home, thought about it, and returned to her doctor to say that she'd had a very good life, was getting on in years, was not afraid of dying, and had decided not to undergo any treatment at all. She asked the doctor to do all he could to make sure she had little or no pain. She lived for several weeks, had enough medication to control the pain, got to the point where she slept on and off most of the day, and slowly and quite happily drifted out of this world into the next. I greatly admired this lady and thought she'd made a good decision. We don't know if we'd have done the same.

In North America the general consensus of orthodox physicians is that cancer should be treated with aggressive measures designed to kill the cancer cells, though the immune system has already failed in its effort to do this. The order of the day is surgery, chemotherapy, and radiation. There are cases where these, singly or in combination, do result in a permanent cure, but this is not what happens in the vast majority of cases. Rather, patients generally experience a considerable amount of pain, disability, and discomfort, after which they are told that they are "in remission." The word "remission" sounds almost like "cure," but before long the tumor is growing again, indicating more chemotherapy, more radiotherapy, more pain and discomfort, and so it goes until, having led a miserable existence for months or years, the patient dies.

In Europe and elsewhere the approach to treating cancer is more gentle. The awesome trio of surgery, chemotherapy, and radiation are used only when other methods have failed, and then only in selected cases. Herbal medicine, naturopathic, homeopathic, osteopathic, anthroposophic medicine, and acupuncture are frequently employed instead, especially in Germany.

Germany has been one of the great innovators in alternative approaches to cancer. German writers say that alternative therapies are safer, more efficacious, and more cost-effective than orthodox methods. The German Medication Law of 1978 gave full legal status to alternative medicines. All German medical students are now taught alternative therapies, and knowledge of these is required for their final examinations. Cancer patients in Germany can thus blend alternative, complementary, and conventional forms of treatment in many ways, and with the blessings of the medical establishment.

Quantum theory reminds us that there are two ways of investigating the properties of light—as waves or as particles. Similarly there are always at least two different ways, and often more, of approaching the problem of diagnosis and treatment of malignant lesions.

Alternate methods of treatment do not often offer a final cancer cure, but they do claim to offer far less debilitating ways of increasing the patient's life-expectancy than chemotherapy, surgery, and radiation. For instance, Dr. Linus Pauling, the winner of two Nobel Prizes, Dr. Ewan Cameron, and their colleagues in California long ago advocated the use of large doses of vitamin C to boost the immune system. They do not say that vitamin C cures cancer, even though there have been cases where patients appeared to be cancer-free years after beginning treatment. But they do claim that vitamin C prolongs life and improves the patient's condition to such an extent that the remaining months or years are comfortable, contented, useful, and satisfying.

Naturopathic physicians have recently taken a prominent place in the treatment of cancer alongside other disciplines that advocate the use of natural herbal remedies. They recommend the use of a multivitamin / mineral complex which includes large doses of vitamin C, selenium, cysteine, co-enzyme Q10, flavonoids, and green tea extracts.

It is difficult to know why so rigid a regime as radiation, surgery, and chemotherapy is advocated so often by North American physicians. It is hard not to suspect that vested interests play a part. We hear that the

CEOs of drug companies that manufacture many of the chemotherapeutic drugs have positions of responsibility on the boards of institutions that treat cancer patients. Many physicians seem chiefly concerned to show that as a result of treatment the size of the tumor has diminished, regardless of the general condition of the patient and of the general state of the patient's life.

There is, however, a growing interest in North America in less drastic methods, with emphasis on mind/body techniques, on spiritual approaches, on adequate doses of vitamins, and on herbal remedies. It seems likely that in the future physicians will increasingly see that cancer is best treated by a combination of orthodox, alternative, and complementary approaches.

What is most harmful in the orthodox attitude toward treatment is that it is often unduly authoritarian and even coercive. We remind ourselves that there is much that is uncertain and unpredictable in the management of cancer, just as there is in almost every sphere of action and in every situation in our world. Many orthodox physicians are unwilling to accept this, though in their hearts they must know that it is true. We need to express more humility, both before the unknown forces behind the disease, and before the often unexplainable factors that go into ameliorating or curing it. Humility would prevent us from laying down the law to our patients and would help us to take time to listen to what they have to say about the management of their problem. The final decision as to what kind of treatment a patient should receive is surely for the patient to make.

The attitude of the physician is important in another respect as well: it can have a material affect on the outcome of the treatment. We have seen how, in quantum theory, there is a close and inevitable connection between the observer and the observed, that the act of observation affects that which is observed, and how in medical treatment the observer and the observed are the physician and the patient. The attitude of the physician colors all that he or she does and influences how the patient feels. How the patient feels about his or her treatment in turn affects the outcome of the treatment. Therefore, if the patient does not feel happy with what the doctor says, how he behaves, or the attitude he takes, the patient should not hesitate to seek help from another doctor.

This may not be an easy thing to do. Often patients come to physicians as to persons with knowledge and authority and do not wish to give up the feeling of security that trust in authority brings. The patient may well be reluctant to make the change to seek help from another doctor. The doctor may resist the idea that the patient should seek help elsewhere, feeling that relinquishing their authority is a relinquishing of responsibility. Generally speaking, in the past patients tended to accept what the doctor said without demur.

The situation today has begun to change. Many patients now demand the right to express their own opinion after hearing what the doctor has to say. The wise physician accepts and indeed welcomes this change and does not raise objections when the patient wants a second opinion or wishes to change to another physician altogether. In fact, a wise physician will often realize that the patient is not entirely happy even before the patient does and will encourage the patient to seek treatment elsewhere.

But things can become very difficult for the patient when he or she has to deal with a trio of surgeon, chemotherapist, and radiotherapist, all of whom have discussed the case in advance and formed a definitive, combined opinion as to the correct form of treatment. Unable to face such an authoritative team, the patient may seek other help without communicating this to the physicians originally concerned. Conflict and tensions result, right where harmony and a positive attitude are what is most required. Nevertheless, it is still really a good sign when a patient is prepared to make the effort to be active on his or her own account, with or without the blessings of the medical authorities. Experience has shown that often the awkward, strong-minded, difficult patient is the one who will do well.

For the reader interested in substantiating many of the views we have expressed in the above paragraphs, we recommend John Robbins's book *Reclaiming Our Health*, which discusses the problem of cancer at great length and provides an extremely well-documented case for much of what we have been saying here.

There are many other problems besides medical ones that a patient faces when diagnosed with cancer. One's financial and psychological well-being are also impacted by the fact of this disease. It is of course often very difficult for a patient to decide what to do or to whom he or she should turn for help and advice, particularly in a problem as "cloudlike" and unpredictable as cancer.

Cloudlike problems do not necessarily require experts to find their solutions. Sometimes wisdom arises through caring communication with loved ones and friends who may have valuable insights, if not of a medical, then of a human kind. Once again, the authoritarian attitude of the experts in an area like cancer, where even today very little is really known, can cause real problems for patients seeking a wise and healthy way to cope with their illness. Often true help can come from a friend, especially if that friend has had cancer or previous experience in this area. A priest, minister, or rabbi may be able to give valuable help. Talking the problem over with husband or wife, with one's children, keeping a channel of communication open with all who are affected by one's being ill, is very, very important.

Frank communication is important, in part, because there are definite healing benefits that come from the loving concern of those who care about you. The care of loved ones, their prayers and healing intentions, can have a marked affect on the well-being and health of the cancer patient. Though this does not on first sight seem to be in the realm of medical practice, there is a real scientific basis for thinking that it is so. There is a profound connection that binds people who share their lives, and that has its basis in physical reality. The interconnectedness that, according to Bell's theorem, is a profound feature of the physical universe is perhaps the most important thing of all in the treatment of cancer.

We recall that, according to this theorem, when two subatomic particles have been in contact and are then separated by a great distance, a change in the "spin" of one will immediately produce a corresponding change in the "spin" of the other. Such togetherness applies equally to human affairs and to the treatment of cancer. There is always a close connection between the patient, the wife or husband, the rest of the family, friends, colleagues, and others concerned (including, last but not least, the physician and those working with him or her).

This kind of close connection has a tremendous effect on the progress of the disease and the recovery from it, through stimulating the immune system. It has been shown in controlled trials that when the wife or husband is loving and supportive, the patient does much better. Group therapy, where patients share their feelings openly, is very effective in maintaining the healthy mental and emotional attitude of the patient.

We have spoken frequently about the "little ripples" that have an adverse effect and the "little nudges" that have a beneficial effect on the individual's physical, mental, and spiritual condition. It is worthwhile to look at these again now. Here once again, very small changes at the beginning of a treatment can have a large effect on the outcome. There are many kinds of such small changes. Patients, their relatives, and others should take advantage of the ripples and nudges we gave in Chapter Two, and regard them as being as important as physical and material approaches to treatment.

One little nudge that is particularly effective is the healing power of laughter! The scientist Norman Cousins, for instance, succeeded in curing himself of a life-threatening rheumatoid illness by administering a stern regimen of abject hilarity: he invited himself to laugh at one thing after another all day long, day after day! He read the funnies and books by comic authors; he listened to comics on the radio, watched humorous videos, with no idea in mind other than to keep himself constantly roaring with laughter. Day by day he got better at laughing and simultaneously regained his health! (Though he did supplement this rigorous therapy with hefty doses of vitamin C.)

While laughter can nudge us into better health, there are other seemingly insignificant details of our existence that can in fact have deleterious consequences. In their book *Dressed to Kill*, Singer and Grismaijer present compelling evidence for a connection between bras and breast cancer in a three-year study of 4,700 women in U.S. cities. The majority who wore their bras more than twelve hours a day but not in bed were twenty-one times more likely to develop breast cancer than those who wore them less than twelve hours a day. Women who wore bras to bed were 125 times more likely to develop breast cancer than those who did not wear them at all.

These findings exemplify the concept from chaos theory that very small irritations can and do lead to large disasters. Here is another example. Recent reports indicate that cancer of the testis is becoming more common. The testis is a very sensitive organ. It is conceivable that tight jeans and close-fitting underwear play a role in the development of this lesion?

Still another little ripple that can lead to cancer is emotional stress, which, as we have mentioned, has an adverse effect on the immune system, making the defense against cancer less efficient. It is common, in looking into the history of a cancer patient, to find that the person was under increased stress at the time when the tumor began to grow. A form of stress that is found frequently to occur in association with the onset of cancer is that due to the loss of a loved one, but any increase in stress, by depressing the immune system, can lead to cancer. It is therefore very important for the patient to deal with this stress, whatever the cause, finding ways of coming to terms with the factors that produce it and encouraging the opposite factors, those that lead to optimism and laughter. This sort of mind / body therapy can often be assisted by friends and family.

Before leaving the subject of the treatment of cancer, we would like to mention a number of books that discuss various aspects of this disease in ways that the layperson can understand. We have already mentioned John Robbins's *Reclaiming Our Health*. Here we would add: *Getting Well Again* by Stephanie and Carl Simonton and James Creighton, which lists the forty-three types of events that commonly lead to stress; *How to Live Longer and Feel Better*, an early classic of alternative medicine by Linus Pauling; *Guide to Alternative Medicine*, an enormously informative encyclopedic survey of the field by Isadore Rosenfeld; *Love, Medicine and Miracles* by Bernie Siegel; *Fighting Disease* by Ellen Michaud and Alice Feinstein; and *Cancer* by John Diamond, Lee Cowden, and Burton

Goldberg. All of the above, going into every aspect of the treatment of cancer, emphasize that one of the most vital things in dealing with cancer is the full and genuine cooperation between orthodox practitioners and those in alternative and complementary medicine.

The new field of psychoneuroimmunology will, in our opinion, be very pertinent to the treatment of cancer in the near future. Future investigation into molecular biology, gene therapy, and genetic engineering should do much to stimulate our interest and bring new ideas and methods to the treatment of cancer. These very important topics are dealt with at length in the chapter "What Causes Cancer" in the book *Cancer* referred to above.

We end this chapter as we began it, by saying that nothing can speak more strongly in favor of our striving for ever-increasing cooperation between orthodox and complementary medicine than the prevention and treatment of cancer. The things we learn from quantum mechanics are the very things we need to put into practice in treating cancer.

# – 15 –

# The Influence of the Home

FROM OUR EARLIER DISCUSSIONS we have come to appreciate the importance of the home and what goes on there between wife, husband, and kids. When a sick person comes to us with a clearcut physical condition, it is often sensible to go ahead and treat him or her without to-do, in a conservative way. When we suspect that all is not well, it is sensible to look to two areas in the patient's environment for the real cause of the problem—the home and the workplace.

If we ask ourselves who in orthodox and complementary medicine is best qualified to assess what goes on in the home, the answer is that a nurse therapist or physician from any discipline can learn to be a sympathetic home visitor. It's a question of being interested in other people and able to put oneself in their shoes. Specialized knowledge and training are important, but intuition is more so. Getting better and feeling better are two complementary aspects of healing.

The respective roles of orthodox and complementary medicine are often reversed. In dealing with the patient who has had a serious operation, the work of the surgeon may be most important and the work of the home visitor complementary. In other instances the physical lesion may be quite minor, and the serious cause of disability may be attributable to something lacking in the home. In this case the task of the home visitor is the major one, and the job of the physician is complementary.

When the sick or injured person has a happy home life, recovery from the majority of accidents and injuries will normally be uneventful. A happy home is worth much more than money and possessions. A poor man's home can be like paradise, a rich man's can be like hell. An intelligent stranger can tell pretty quickly when he's a visitor in a happy home. Like a roaring log fire on a cold winter day, the ambience of a happy home cheers one as soon as one gets through the door. A home where there is unhappiness can be a chilling experience for the visitor

Starting a home begins with two people attracted to one another, committed to one another, deriving pleasure from being together, treating one another in a loving manner, with consideration, kindness, and respect. It is essential for a husband and wife to appreciate the extreme importance of a healthy sexual relationship. It is good that both partners learn from one another frankly and openly how they feel about making love, giving each other the maximum amount of pleasure in the process, understanding each one's little foibles. This act involves both mind and body, both sex organs and the whole of the body. It is good for the man to be prepared to hold back until he's sure his wife is going to be satisfied. Without this relationship, which calls for a good deal of hard work, the life of the home and family can be jeopardized, and personal problems can develop that affect mental, spiritual, and physical health.

Just as in quantum mechanics, it's the little nudges that make all the difference. One should refrain from laughing at peculiar ideas and feelings from the other partner. Loving attention from the spouse is often the most important therapy for a stressful day at work. These are all things that the visiting nurse or physician has to bear in mind when visiting the home. The man who's stressed after a tough day at the office, fed up with his work, disappointed because things aren't going well, or depressed because he's out of work can get a lot of help from his wife, and vice versa. Sex is a good way to mutual understanding. It can tell a man that his wife thinks a lot of him, admires him, relies on him, and this gives him back his self respect. As for the wife who's had a tough day at home, feeling off color, irritated by the kids, loving attention from the husband makes all the difference to her life.

When the husband and wife are on the same wavelength, they can build a very happy home. The visitor from outside experiences at once the warmth and sunshine of that home. Not only do husband and wife support one another, but their kids have the best chance of growing up to be contented, solid citizens. A spirit of togetherness between wife and husband produces a feeling of significance and security, not only for them but for the children as well. When there's strife in the home, husband and wife are much more prone to minor accidents that lead to one or the other becoming an injured worker. It's not difficult for the stranger visiting such a home to detect that there's strife there. A prospective double-blind study was carried out in the United States some years ago on male patients who'd had a heart attack. The group in which the wives showed them love and affection made a better recovery than the group of men without this extra attention.

These are things that should go through the mind of the physician when he first sees the sick patient in his office or the worker who's hurt himself at work. A few questions can make the doctor suspect that all is not well in the home. Quite often he or she can do a lot to remedy this. When in doubt, it's good to call the psychologist.

I (WHK-W) recall the case of a young man who presented with symptoms and signs that suggested the existence of a cauda equina syndrome, but the picture was not quite right. Fortunately I called in a sympathetic psychologist, who discovered the cause of this man's severe disability. His mother-in-law had been living with him and his wife on the farm. For a variety of reasons the young man found her intolerable, and his symptoms stemmed from this. He couldn't stand it any longer. Speedy arrangements were made for the mother-in-law to take a long holiday far from her daughter and son-in-law. The man made an almost instantaneous recovery, much to my surprise and relief. So instead of hours spent in the operating room I had time for a mug or two of beer with my psychologist friend.

It is always good in the case of an injured worker to talk to the spouse and bring him or her into the picture. It's better still to visit the home. A spouse with the right attitude can do as much and sometimes more than anyone else to help his or her mate, as much with problems at work as with those in the home. It takes a lot of practice and sympathetic understanding on the doctor's part when talking to the other spouse about this kind of situation.

What we've seen in our travels has convinced us that a happy home life is considered vital throughout the world. One wonders how king Solomon managed with all those wives and concubines, not to mention the horses and chariots! Was he all that wise after all? In some countries the woman has no say in things that affect her home, life, and welfare. They are nothing more than chattels at the beck and command of their husbands, which is of course an appalling state of affairs.

We've stressed the effect that small, apparently unimportant things have on the relations between husband and wife. It's the same way with the relations between fellows of colleges and undergrads and between bosses and people working for them. We simply don't give adequate attention to these little things; often they just don't occur to us. Some years ago one of our freshmen at university committed suicide. Perhaps we couldn't have done anything, but we blamed ourselves for not being perceptive enough to see that something was very much wrong.

In summary, there are two things we'd like to emphasize: When a sick or injured person isn't getting better quickly, look into affairs in the home. This brings all disciplines in complementary medicine close together, for a member of any one can, with careful training, take on the job of gently probing what goes on in the home. This is a job that is really complementary to every other kind of medical practice, conventional and alternative.

# — 16 —

# The Workplace

WE BELIEVE THAT THE CONNECTION between the affairs of the workplace and those of complementary medicine is a close one. This is an extremely important area, and one in which there is unlimited scope for any physician or therapist with sufficient interest to acquire the necessary skill and ability to succeed.

It is said that the gods like the taste of salt: the sweat of human effort is the savor of their sacrifices. In recent years there has been a marked increase in human effort in the attempt to prevent and relieve disability from work-related low back pain, as discussed by Frank and six colleagues in the *Canadian Medical Association Journal* of June 16, 1998. In their presentation they suggest that management during the first four weeks should be conservative. Studies that focus on return to work, implemented in the subacute stage, show reductions in time lost of thirty to fifty percent following adequately planned treatment. They say there is evidence that employers who are prepared to modify the patient's duties in the workplace can reduce time lost by at least thirty percent. On a slightly different tack they suggest that a combination of several different approaches in a workplace-linked system can produce a fifty-percent reduction in time lost at no extra cost and even in some cases with significant savings.

These writers condemn piecemeal approaches and conclude by saying that only by engaging all those with a common stake in the issue, physicians, nurses, managers at work, rehabilitation experts, and insurers, among others, and by obtaining active collaboration of all of them, can this important cause of disability be controlled in our time.

The ambience of the workplace is as important as that of the home in maintaining the health and contentment of the worker. The individual who works for him or herself is seldom incapacitated for long by injury to the point where he or she is unable to work. Such a person has a strong incentive to continue at work. The self-employed person can make the necessary adaptation to compensate for the disability. These are two vitally important things, and we have to bear them in mind when considering the factors that make it much more difficult for the employee to remain at work or get back to work after an injury.

Nortin Hadler, writing in the *New England Journal of Medicine* of July 31, 1997, wrote, "Rather than focusing on ergonomic remedies, we should guarantee workplaces that are comfortable when we are well and accommodating when we are ill. . . . When one or more workers find their musculoskeletal discomfort intolerable or incapacitating, we should not impugn their veracity. Rather we should question just what in the workplace is compromising their ability to cope. Consideration of styles of management, job security, and group dynamics is far more likely to help the injured person than another exercise in ergonometrics."

The attitudes of managers in a business or factory set the stage for the way in which the actors, the workers, perform. The CEO who is efficient, hard-working, and considerate of his workers is the one who will develop and maintain a profitable business. It's not difficult to pick out the good manager. Roger Ackhoff, a well-known management consultant, is of the opinion that the CEO has no easy task. Problems and difficulties do not come singly. The manager has to deal with an infinite variety of combinations of interlocking problems. Ackhoff says the job of the successful CEO is not to manage problems but to deal with a "mess" (R.

Ackhoff, "Reflections on the Hawthorne Effect" in the *Chiropractic Report*, vol. 14, no. 1, 1989). He should spend more time on the floor than in his office, which should be in a place as accessible as possible to everyone.

In some organizations, a hospital for example, the CEO and staff of assistants conceal themselves in a palatial office on the top floor, far from the activity of wards, outpatient departments, and operating rooms. Superficially such a peaceful, comfortable environment makes life easier for the administrators, but in the long run problems catch up with them, they become out of touch with the activities of the institution, and the hospital or other concern becomes an inefficient one. In such a setting the doctors in the hospital or stewards on the shop floor and then the workers themselves begin to realize that their bosses are not interested in getting alongside them. The CEO's assistant managers and their secretarial staff take their cue from him. When they see he's concerned with the welfare of the workers, they are likely to develop the same sort of interest too. The workers in turn take their cue from the shop stewards.

In their small and fascinating monograph *The One-Minute Manager*, K. Blanchard, Ph.D. and S. Johnson, M.D. discuss, in a most entertaining way, the qualities desirable in a business manager: clear understanding of his aims and objectives expressed in one-minute goals: one-minute praisings to the workers for jobs well done and one-minute reprimands for jobs not well done. Reprimands can be made gently, as for example, "I'm surprised that a reliable worker like you could do . . ." Their aim, of course, is to suggest how a man or woman studying to be a manager can become a good one. The Mayo brothers in their clinic in Rochester, Minnesota, were getting at the same thing when, in teaching their residents in surgery, they said that two pats on the back to one kick in the pants is in the right proportion. And this long before the days of management consultants!

Senior administrators are by no means always efficient, hard-working, and kindly. Some are blustering bullies concerned only with their own advancement. Some are lazy. Some are unintelligent. Some are not prepared to face up to the problems that are bound to arise from time to time. At one stage, as head of a hospital department, I (WHK-W) worked under a chief executive who listened to what I had to say, and promised to think about it and get back to me in a week or so—but he never did. I had but little respect for him.

In another job I worked for a senior surgeon who was wise enough never to take on more than three new problems at any one time. I learned to bide my time when my request was turned down, hoping that if I repeated the request a week or two later, I'd get the boss when he only had one or two problems on his plate. This same surgeon often used to say, "I'll think about your suggestion." If I was lucky I'd find three weeks later that the boss had accepted my idea as his own. We both participated in these games with mutual enjoyment, pretending we didn't understand what the other was getting at! Heads of departments, shop stewards, head nurses, and others in positions of responsibility, just like the boss, are good, bad, and indifferent. Fortunate indeed is the worker whose boss has a kindly sense of humor, as mine did.

Intelligent, keen CEOs spend a lot of time wandering round the floor, listening, looking around, asking questions. They have their assistants do the same thing. It's much better to have meetings with the stewards or department heads and with the workers in a corner somewhere on the floor, where the action is, than up in the executive office. Informal meetings are much more effective than formal ones. It's good to find out from the men and women how they're getting on with their work, what they feel about it, what problems they have and what criticisms. It's helpful to know them by name and be able to ask them about things at home. The stewards should report in confidence any troubles a worker has. This enables CEOs to know and show that they know about people's problems. Good managers don't mind a few critical comments. They appreciate suggestions from the people actually doing the work. The workers, for their part, come to appreciate the manager's interest in them as people as well as in their work.

It's important for CEOs to talk about the goals they set their people. It should be possible for them to set these down on paper quite briefly, in a page or so. All this gives CEOs the chance to make sure that the workers understand what is required from them for the factory's efficiency and to correct them when they haven't got the picture right. Then they are all on the same wavelength. This should be done in a pleasant way, taking care not to appear critical. As CEOs wander round they look for the chance of congratulating people who are doing a good job. When they spot a man or woman doing a shoddy job, they say something like this: "I'm surprised and disappointed to see an efficient, trustworthy person like you turning out second-class work. You usually do such good work." This is, of course, William Mayo's "two pats on the back to one kick in the pants!" And it works. These little things—the nudges—help CEOs take individuals and train them to make a team.

The ancient Greeks used to put these very same ideas into practice during the Olympic, Doric, and Ionic Games. This is well expressed in Wilder Penfield's book *The Torch*, written about Hippocrates' life and times. The prize for the winner of a race was a laurel wreath, which went with the kudos the athlete obtained. Winners gave back their laurel wreaths to the god Apollo. Winners of the triathlon, the three-part race, gave the golden tripod with which they were rewarded to Apollo, too. Somewhat surprisingly many workers today are equally rewarded by praise and encouragement for their work. It's good to have some symbol like the laurel wreath. On the North American continent today citizens are beginning to move back to emphasis on responsibilities rather than solely on rights.

The work environment is something quite vital. It is the CEO who does most to determine what it's like. Among other things it is important that the individual worker have adequate working space and not be cramped. There must be adequate lighting, heat, and fresh air. Some years ago the manager of Western Electric in the United States brought in a firm of consultants, industrial psychologists and others, to suggest and institute improvements to the factory floor. Among other things, they thought the lighting was inadequate. They told the workers that they were going to do something about this and increased the intensity of the lighting to a marked degree. The output from each worker increased to a corresponding degree. One of the psychologists suggested a further experiment to prove that it really was the increased lighting that was responsible for the improved output of the workers.

The consultants then called the workers together and told them they were going to make further changes, giving the impression that they were going to increase the intensity of the lighting still further. In fact they decreased it considerably. The output of the workers then again increased to a marked degree, demonstrating that it was the interest shown in the workers that was responsible for more productive work and not the lighting at all.

To show interest in the welfare of the worker is probably more important than anything else. In well-run concerns, CEOs have frequent meetings with their staffs, with floor stewards, and with the men and women under them. On occasion CEOs meet with all the workers. This pays good dividends. Provided that a boss gives workers time to air their opinions, including their complaints, while she listens carefully, she can often then make her own decisions, incorporating only some of the workers' suggestions. To be consulted is often more important than to have a say in the decision-making process. In an earlier chapter we saw how important it is to listen patiently and to show interest. The ideal of course is to run the plant so that workers feel they are part of a happy family. No one says this is an easy task.

Some years ago I (WHK-W) copied the clever ploy of the Campbell Clinic in Memphis, Tennessee, in a Canadian orthopedic department. In this clinic there was a weekly meeting of the surgical staff and their residents to discuss the treatment of their patients. There was a free-for-all at the end of the meeting, during which anyone, senior or junior, could say anything they liked, however uncomplimentary. The chief didn't mind being criticized by a junior resident. But only during this half hour! Usually the comments were accompanied by a good deal of laughter. I found this worked well for me in Saskatoon. It was good to give the chaps a chance of letting off steam once a week. Quite often there'd be an idea that was really good. Sometimes the chairman would say, "That's been tried already, and it didn't work." It was more important to let people say what was on their minds than to accept their suggestion.

So far we have talked about abstract rewards, which are most important and effective. We turn now to consider practical, material rewards. Good work should be rewarded by a raise in salary before the worker demands it. A young clerk in a business office in Melbourne was offered a better-paid job in another firm. He went to tell his boss that he was leaving for this reason. The boss said, "If you stay with us, we'll be prepared to give you a raise here right now." The young clerk asked, "Do you really think I'm worth it?" "Yes we do," replied the boss. "Then I'm leaving," said the clerk. "I don't want to work for people who don't acknowledge my worth till driven to it." That young man became a bishop! And he treated clergy and others under his authority as he wanted to be treated himself.

A yearly bonus for good work done for a business concern that has made a profit is another good ploy. The worker is discouraged when he sees that the upper echelons in large institutions and other concerns get immense increases in salary and she does not get any at all. This unfortunate situation seems, from reading the press, to be the case with some of our large banks and with other large concerns, too. Better still is the system sometimes adopted of making it possible for workers to have shares in the business and thus be stimulated to work hard for that business in order to share in the profits themselves. It is good that workers see that there are chances of promotion for work well done and responsibilities well shouldered.

The things we have been discussing all go to make an ideal business or factory environment in which there is a much-reduced possibility of workers suffering injury, and if the worker is injured a much greater chance of getting him or her back to work quickly. The writers do not presume to pontificate by saying that every CEO and his or her staff are expected to subscribe to all the conditions for good business mentioned above. We have come across nearly all of them in one business or another and have heard about others, not only in America, but in Europe and the East as well. The greater the number of these criteria any concern can meet, the greater the chance of getting the injured worker back to work quickly.

The things we have talked about in discussing the work of the CEO apply equally to those at all subordinate managers and junior staff. In fact, faults in leadership may be encountered more often in this group, and it may require great tact to persuade members of the group to alter their habits.

The reader may be tempted to assume that the attitudes and the abilities of the managers is the only factor to be considered in defining the attributes of the "good" business concern. This is far from being our intention. Wise managers deal with unsatisfactory workers along the lines of *The One-Minute Manager*. Most workers do respond to one-minute praising and one-minute reprimands, but of course there are workers who fail to respond to these measures. How does the manager deal with the individual whose work is putting the whole business concern into jeopardy? It is wise to have groups of three or four workers, senior and junior, whom one can trust to deal with such a situation, especially when it is a question of sacking a person, both for their advice and for their help in dealing with the offender. We all know that serious disruptions and even strikes of the workers can arise from apparently small individual incidents. The "little ripples" we encounter in chaos theory reminds us of this.

Dr. Dale Mierau of the Saskatoon Interdisciplinary Musculoskeletal Centre writes, "There is great value in having the therapist visit the workplace of the injured worker to assess the situation for him or herself. This costs money and is time-consuming but saves much suffering and high costs in the long run. The workplace is used for a graduated return to work, a part of the rehabilitation process, or we could say as an adjunct to the clinic, to simulate the duties, environment, and demands of the workplace and thus limit the time away from work—in other words to keep the injured worker in the workplace all the time till he or she is better.

"This graduated return to work is done with the insurer providing a full-time income to the worker, so that he or she has few financial worries, and so that the employer is not out-of-pocket or short-staffed. The replacement worker, someone doing the job temporarily, is paid a full salary as well. When the injured worker is fit for work again, the services of the replacement worker are terminated, and the injured worker resumes work again on full pay. A convenient source of supply for a replacement worker is from the list of people recently retired. The insuring agency has to bear the cost of paying the salaries of both injured worker and the replacement, which is more expensive in the short run but very much less costly in the long run.

"This plan involves cooperation between worker, employer, insurer, family doctor, and those undertaking the rehabilitation. The people who provide the rehabilitation do not get involved with disputes and disagreements. These are handled by others, so that the provider though retaining autonomy remains neutral." We guess the secret is for the chap in charge, Dale Mierau in this case, to convince the insurer who pays the bill that he can deliver the goods.

A similar approach was used forty years ago by Dr. Plewes, an orthopedic surgeon in Luton, England, who cooperated with the managers and shop stewards on the floor of the Vauxhall car factory in that town. Plewes and his staff actually visited the plant regularly to assess the patient's progress and prescribe treatment. The results were excellent. Plewes was a good actor, and that helped him to convince his audience. He was far ahead of his time. This approach fits in with what Dr. Nortin Hadler has to say, that when the injured worker fails to return to work in a reasonable length of time, we should not impugn his veracity but rather question how the set up in the workplace is compromising his ability to work—and do something about it!

The key to such a scheme, pioneered by Dr. Plewes in England in the 1950s and recently carried some steps further by Dr. Mierau, is cooperation between the visitor from the multidisciplinary clinic and the staff of the workplace. This calls for special qualities from special people. The visitor's first job is to get alongside the staff of the business concern or factory, so that he or she is readily accepted by them. It's another one of those jobs that involve patience, starting slowly, and moving ahead gradually. The ability to feel at ease with CEOs, department head managers, shop stewards, foremen, and workers is essential. By no means does every would-be visitor have this ability.

He or she must also know how to assess the things that take place in the workplace day by day. We have dealt with many of these things in the first part of this chapter. Quite quickly the experienced visitor can see the strong and the weak points about any workplace. In addition, he or she has to know how to keep quiet about the things noticed. The art is to know how to talk to the CEO and others without irritating them. The advice of *the One-Minute Manager* helps here.

It's a good ploy to talk about the things that are going well and quietly congratulate the manager before tackling difficult matters, at first in a very tentative way. When rapport has been established, confidence soon follows, and both sides can feel happy and be frank with each other. The visitor should be a professional with the expertise to investigate and deal with problems between managers and the injured worker as well as difficulties, physical and psychological, experienced by the worker. Joint decisions have to be made with regard to the patient's progress and ability to progress to more active and heavier work.

Dr. Andrew Clarke of Ontario Heath and Safety writes that it is the kind of relationship a man or woman has with his or her work that most strongly affects the tendency to leave work or remain off duty when there is a problem such as an injury at work. Work disability in many cases is a psychological or behavioral issue and not a medical one. Job security is not really an incentive to return to work; rather lack of security is a disincentive. The conditions that are currently the source of increasing amounts of disability in society all have one thing in common—uncertainty. He goes on to say that clearly the most effective intervention one can make in helping an injured worker back to work is to invite that worker to the workplace for a meeting specifically about return to work. The manager or employer must then make a real effort to make sure that this meeting conveys welcome and supportiveness to the worker, including a concrete offer of modified work, if at all possible.

Few of us appreciate the benefit that accrues when a physician learns to combine two different jobs. We first noticed this in Professor James in the Orthopedic Department of Edinburgh University. His clinical work was divided between spine and hand surgery. This struck us as rather odd. In talking to him we realized that the shift from one type of operating to another was relaxing for him. It's good for the administrator who spends a lot of time at his desk to have tasks that take him round the factory to meet and talk with the workers. It's equally good for the surgeon to have tasks that involve time at his desk.

The majority of chiropractors spend their day treating one patient after another. It's good that some of them, not all, like being a member of a team such as Dr. Mierau's, and that people like Dr. Lubcke in Portland get a kick out of building a multidisciplinary team. His consists of one family practitioner, one medical internist, one osteopath, one nurse practitioner, three chiropractors, one acupuncturist, and one social worker to form a general health care clinic.

Many such clinics are springing up hither and yon, and it will be good in days to come to find people of an equally diverse group taking an interest in becoming expert visitors to different workplaces. There is abundant room for this kind of person, chosen from internists, family practitioners, chiropractors, acupuncturists, and all the other disciplines in complementary medicine. John Bell, with his theory of togetherness, would remind us that we are all closely interconnected. In the past doctors other than those in mainstream medicine have felt left out in the cold. They need to remember that orthodox doctors also have felt that their services were not appreciated, especially by their patients. To appreciate this encourages all of us to make the effort to work together.

We do well to remember what Nortin Hadler has said, that the workplace, small or large, should be comfortable when we are well and accommodating when we are ill. We physicians, of whatever discipline, must learn to feel comfortable when working for the patient's good with physicians of other disciplines and to be accommodating as well.

At this point it might be helpful to picture a discussion along the following lines:

*Dr. Kirke:* It is true that most people are content when they feel the boss listens to them and is interested in their opinion. This matters more than trying to satisfy everyone, an impossibility. The CEO can take back to his office all the comments made in the meeting and try to synthesize them into what he thinks workable.

*Visitor (a historian):* It's noteworthy that twenty years ago we all thought that Japan had the edge on us in the practical use of technology, and now we see that Japan as a country has overreached itself. Political leaders got carried away by success and forgot to regulate the banks. Of course in the modern world regulations do stifle initiative, but we do need to give some thought to regulations. It's difficult to have a balanced approach.

*Visitor (an economist):* Knowing how to deal with the unsatisfactory worker must be one of the greatest difficulties. I get your point that it's helpful to obtain the advice of a chap's fellow workers. Often the union has to be consulted. Can one say to the union official, "I'm disappointed that a union as reliable as yours condones poor work in one of your members?" The "one-minute reprimand" approach?

*Dr. Kirke:* The support of coworkers and of union officials is very important. We should use their help more often.

Visitor: It must be tricky, something quite difficult, to get the right sort of person, often a nurse I think you said, to sort things out in the workplace. The wrong sort of visitor could so easily get the back up of the CEO and the people working for him.

*Dr. Kirke:* You're right. The wrong kind of visitor could do more harm than good. The best way of training someone to be a factory or plant visitor is to apprentice him or her to someone already known to be the right sort of person for this job. This can only be accomplished by personal contact and teaching on the spot.

In summary, we'd like to emphasize two things: (1) Anyone with the right attitude can learn to be an effective plant visitor. Here is real scope for many in complementary medicine. Anyone who's prepared to learn can do this. Often we look for the nurse to be trained for this job. We'd like to see some chiropractors, massage therapists, physical therapists, and psychologists, among others, prepared to be visitors to the plant. The physician or surgeon in orthodox medicine may well be at a disadvantage, simply because he or she is accustomed to think so much about blood tests, X ray and MRI results, and so on, that often it's difficult to find time and energy for treating patients as people. (2) The combination of patience and tact, of enjoying interacting with people, are the really essential qualities.

# – 17 –

# The Nurse

THE ORIGIN OF THE PROFESSION of nursing goes back thousands of years, certainly to between 2000 and 3000 B.C. The Greek priest-esses and the priests undoubtedly combined nursing care for the suppli-ants with their sacred duties at the temple of Apollo at Delphi as well as in the temples at Corinth and Epidauros. These glamorous young men and women served the shrine, took part in healing for the sick, and also were on call as prostitutes. In Corinth at one time there were more than a thousand sacred prostitutes who served the temples of Asclepius and Aphrodite. Nurses today need not be disturbed to learn that their noble profession had such origins, for there has always been a deep connection between religion and sex. It is as strong as ever today. Doctors and other health workers had a very similar origin.

Throughout Europe in the Middle Ages the monasteries for men and convents for women included healing in their work for the poor and needy. Monks and nuns, lay brothers and sisters, were very much involved in collecting, preparing, and administering herbs to the sick who came to them for help. They prepared herbs and other natural products in a shed called a herbarium. The nursing of the sick and aged in the infir-maries was under the care and supervision of these lay brothers and sisters, as we read in Ellis Peters' Cadfael stories. In later centuries, and particularly in Britain after Henry VIII dissolved the monasteries, much of the care of the sick, which of course included nursing, was no longer subject to monastic discipline, and the standards of care distinctly deteriorated. It wasn't until the nineteenth century that medical standards took a clear turn for the better, and nursing was in the vanguard of this improvement. During the Crimean War in Europe, Florence Nightingale worked hard to persuade the military authorities to allow her to improve the standard of nursing of the wounded. The result of her work was greatly improved hygiene and a fall in the mortality rate for injured soldiers from forty to just two percent. In Britain, and more widely as well, she is acknowledged with awe as the founder of modern nursing. With her work nursing as a profession had come into its own.

In the United States trained nurses were an unknown quantity before 1870. The care of sick people was committed to lower-class women conscripted from penitentiaries and almshouses. Little attention was given to cleanliness and hygiene. The reform of nursing was undertaken by upper-class women who, following the lead of Florence Nightingale, became the guardians of a new hygienic order, working in state charities' Aid Associations from 1872 on. Some doctors appreciated the work of these highly educated women and supported them in their desire to establish nurses' training schools. The development of such schools was to revolutionize medical practice by providing a large cadre of well-trained women to provide medical care where it was needed but where the constant attention of a fully qualified physician was not required.

There were many physicians at the time, however, who vehemently opposed these newcomers to their medical turf, observing that educated nurses would not "do as they were told"! But the reformers went over the heads of the doctors. They used their own social status to gain the aid of powerful men of their own class, very much aware, no doubt, that Florence Nightingale had done the same thing, finding allies in the high places of the British government. As with so many other improvements in the history of medicine, it was people outside of the medical establishment who in fact did the work to establish nursing as a profession. Soon physicians came to rely on the new kind of nurses and many schools for nursing were founded. There were only three such schools in 1873, but there were 432 by 1900 and 1,129 by 1910.

By 1902 nurses were deeply engaged in public health activities in New York, visiting schools, referring children to physicians, speaking to parents, treating minor conditions, teaching self care, and doing follow-up work. Nurses were strongly established as anesthetists by 1920. By 1930 recognition was given to three kinds of nurses: registered nurses, licensed practical nurses, and nursing aides. Though there were many circumstances such as poor neighborhoods, rural areas, undeveloped countries where physicians were very scarce, and where a well-trained nurse would be perfectly capable of performing such routine functions as diagnosis and referral, nurses were not permitted to perform these services. They were clearly subordinate to physicians and were kept in a position of dependence upon them.

By middle of the twentieth century the medical world had, however, become quite dependent on nurses, but increasingly qualified nurses were in short supply. By 1960 it had become a crisis, particularly in America, and health care suffered. Fortunately, shortly after that the situation improved, and nursing care took a leap forward. In the conflicts of the 1970s nurses allied themselves with consumers, so that the doctors and hospitals ceased to dominate the scene as completely as they had in the past.

At the present time the basic training for a registered nurse is four years for the degree program. The trainee, on passing the final examination, is licensed as a Registered Nurse (R.N.) with a Bachelor of Science degree. A further two years of training is required for the degree of Master of Science. In Canada it is usual for those seeking work as a community health nurse, a nurse in administration, or a nurse in education to have this higher degree. In the United States, the Canadian B.S. is recognized as being more practically oriented than the B.S. in the United States, and some with this degree can apply for jobs normally requiring an M.S. The pressure these days is to get a Bachelor of Nursing qualifying degree, with State Registration. For the master's degree nurses are usually encouraged to take a clinical specialty or community nursing or education. Some go on to take a Ph.D. degree.

A recent trend in the United States, that is of concern to physicians, allows the entry into medical practice of a variety of nonmedical professionals. In 1998 the National Public Radio program "All Things Considered " discussed the changing role of advanced-practice nurses in health care. This discussion centered around the work of the Columbia Advanced Practice Nurse Association of the Columbia School of Nursing in New York. The Presbyterian Hospital asked for help from the nursing school in providing health care in poor neighborhoods in Manhattan. In return for this the hospital agreed to grant the nursing school two primary care practices with admitting privileges to the wards. One of these was to be with physicians and nurse practitioners working as equals, and the other was to be entirely run by nurse practitioners alone. A short while later the Oxford Health Plan and some other HMO providers in New York City adopted a similar plan, granting nurse practitioners freedom to practice along the lines of physicians; they could diagnose, treat, refer, and bill for services as medical doctors do. We understand that nurse practitioners in other states have been granted similar privileges and it appears likely that this will spread quite quickly across North America.

As one would expect, the doctors have their questions. Even if medical standards are comparable to those provided by physicians, will patient satisfaction with treatment by nurses be as great as that from physicians? Will all insuring agencies be satisfied? For nurse practitioners the basic issue is, indeed, insurance coverage, i.e., that patients be covered for receiving primary care from nurse practitioners. It is of interest to note that the amount of freedom given to nurses at present varies a great deal according to circumstances.

In sparsely populated areas in North America, especially in the far north where doctors are thin on the ground, much greater scope is afforded to the nurse. In Africa and in the East medical care is often grossly inadequate. I (WHK-W) was for a number of years the only surgeon doing mainly orthopedic work between Cairo and Johannesburg. In district hospitals in Kenya of a hundred beds, there were often 150 to 200 inpatients, many lying on mats between the beds. One doctor had to administer the hospital, give medical, surgical, and obstetric care, look after the finances, pay regular visits to outlying dispensaries, and act as the medical officer of health to a large district. While the doctor was "on safari" most if not all so-called medical duties had to be done by nurses, and they were usually very well done. When the doctor was at home, medical and nursing duties were often shared.

I recall an amusing incident that took place in a small government hospital. The senior doctor was no surgeon. His assistant, newly qualified, had little surgical skill. The one nurse on the hospital staff had spent several years in charge of the operating room of the large central hospital. On this occasion it was obvious to the young doctor that the African woman in labor required an urgent cesarian section. He and the nurse scrubbed up. An African assistant nurse gave the anesthetic. The doctor did the actual cutting, instructed by the nurse at every step. When he was really stuck, the nurse made a deft move or two with scissors or scalpel, and then handed the instrument back to him! Mother and baby did splendidly. Throughout the country this was no solitary instance of such mutual cooperation. The point is that in situations where fully qualified physicians are scarce, often nurses are the best resource for saving lives.

At the present time in North America we look to nurses to fulfill a number of functions, and this is increasing. Many nurses are most competent administrators. They play an important role in the realm of public health. They do well as educators They are a valuable adjunct to the doctor's office. We now look to them, both female and male nurses, for help when we think that there are problems in the home or in the workplace. These are very important and sensitive areas that call for help from a person who has great understanding of people and their relationships to one another. There should be no problem for a nurse to handle any reasonable situation.

Nurses today must be able to handle a complexity of human relation situations, such as staffing levels and ever-changing technologies and skills, union requirements for a variety of unions, politics of varying levels, and the usual patient/family/community issues. In addition the nurse must have the personal capabilities to handle many kinds of stress, such as heavy workloads, reduced staffing, frequent reorganization, demands from many different levels, and family responsibilities.

The introduction of the nurse case manager into the Workers' Compensation setting has been an improvement in a situation where there has been a lack of communication among the principal parties, including the employer, payer, health care providers, and the patient. Nurses serve as an intermediary among the parties involved. The process, which has in the past frequently been slow, inefficient, and costly, is expedited, resulting in greater efficiency at a lower cost. The nurse case manager frequently accompanies the patient to the doctor's office and offers the doctor the opportunity to discuss the clinical issues in the case in a direct manner. This saves the doctor and his or her staff a great deal of time and difficulty in obtaining authorization for any additional diagnostic testing or treatment, if it seems appropriate. Issues of returning to modified work and later to regular work are also discussed in this setting, which is an advantage to all concerned.

There's room for a lot more study here. The same type of situation arises when there are difficulties in the workplace. The nurse who goes into the place of work to help solve a personal problem has to be sensitive not only to the sick man or woman but to the other workers, the shop steward or other supervisor, CEO, and representative of the insurer. For these two activities alone, we're going to be asking much more of the nurse in days to come.

We're sure it's not out of place to end this important discussion in a lighter vein. During the Victorian era in Britain the hospital matron, the director of nursing, was an individual with great authority and unlimited prestige. Miss Luckes, matron of the London Hospital, was accustomed to drive around her district each afternoon in her splendid, double-horse-drawn carriage. The matron of St. Bartholomew's Hospital was a friend of my (WHK-W) family. She used to confide in my parents, telling them how terrifying she found the staff men, the physicians, and the surgeons. Many years later I met the senior surgeon of St. Bartholomew's who, during discussion of hospital affairs, admitted that the same matron was a terror to all concerned!

During the second World War a friend of mine, a resident in obstetrics and gynecology, married a charming young lady whom he'd met in that department. He joined the army, and during the course of the required exercises he had to learn to descend in a parachute. On the last occasion he made a poor landing, injured his knees, and was laid up for several weeks. His wife asked the matron for two weeks leave to nurse her husband. "Never heard of such nonsense," said the matron. "But last week, matron, you gave Nurse Jones two weeks leave to nurse her mother," replied the young nurse, showing great daring. The matron replied, "Remember nurse, mothers are essential; husbands are not." In the end the matron met her Waterloo. She married the chairman of the board of governors of the local brewery!

Nurses will continue to occupy a position of great importance in the delivery of health care. Healing is a God-given gift, and the nursing profession has been exemplary in this respect.

# – 18 –

# Listening and Asking

TWO OF THE MOST valuable tools doctors have at their disposal for helping the patient toward recovery are the ability to listen to what the patient has to say and then to ask the patient what he or she thinks, rather than say right away what we think should be done. We have talked about the various nudges that are effective. These are two of them that become even more effective when the patient can see that the doctor is really interested in their thoughts.

The ability to listen is something that every physician and therapist can acquire. Without it we cannot expect to help any of our patients. We often think that the aromatherapist or the massage therapist or chiropractor has an advantage over the orthodox physician, because he or she doesn't have to spend time and energy thinking about complex technical equipment and so can concentrate on this essential art. That doesn't excuse any one of us from finding time to listen. When at a loss for time or energy at the end of a busy day, it is sensible to schedule another appointment when we have adequate time and are relaxed enough to give our attention to what the patient has to tell us.

Dr. Bernard Lown, cardiologist and Nobel Prize winner, as reported in the *Boston Globe Magazine* of October 13, 1996, believes that it is often necessary for the physician to spend an hour with the patient to develop rapport with him or her. The usual fifteen minutes with each patient prescribed by the paying agency is often not enough. One of the most important ingredients is the spending of time, something many of us are loathe to do. "The chief complaint of the patient is often no more than an admission ticket to the doctor," says Dr. Lown.

Frequently the things that the patient says are bothering him turn out to be irrelevant. The physical complaint is often the tip of the iceberg, the tip of a much larger personal problem. It is not possible in every case to delve deeply into mental, emotional, and social problems. Experience is in the long run the best guide as to when the patient's situation calls for an all-out effort. It is experience also that helps and guides the doctor in balancing the needs of each patient and the demands made by time in the long and busy day.

The art of listening is a complex one. Fifty years ago medical students were taught to listen to the heart and lungs with a stethoscope, something intriguing for the neophyte. Now, something more fascinating, we learn to listen to the whole patient with ears, eyes, and something akin to extrasensory perception. Dr. Lown dares to say that if the physician cannot assess seventy-five percent of what goes on in the patient's mind when he has finished listening, he should go back to medical school.

In the practice of medicine today it is most important to uphold the role of "evidence-based" medicine. Dr. Lown points out that much of medicine, as a healing art that relies on a unique bond between two or more human beings (pure quantum), "depends profoundly on science, though it is not a science." In the work of healing, as in other areas, we are compelled to realize that the nature of our world is a combination of the Newtonian and the quantum approach. In practice this means that while we are striving to be scientific, there is still a lot of room for the exercise of intuition. After all we all have a brain with a left and a right side to it, the left logical and the right intuitive. The whole person exercises both.

We learned that it was only after many years of practice that we began to appreciate the value of listening. In earlier years I (WHK-W) was impressed by an account of an Austrian physician who ran a private clinic for individuals from all over Europe who were suffering from stress and emotional strain as well as from physical exhaustion. After listening attentively for as long as necessary, he used to nod his head and quietly pronounce the one German word *Zo*. Nothing he heard ever surprised him. There was no hint of disparagement in his voice and manner. This was encouraging to many, many sick people who learned to trust him and open their hearts with confidence. We can read elsewhere about other doctors who have learned the same lesson. I certainly was not intelligent enough to get the message myself for many years.

My teacher was a dirty, ill-kempt, overweight, garrulous man of about fifty. He came into my office at the end of a long clinic on a Friday afternoon. Something told me at once that here was a person I could do nothing to help. My chief concern was to escape as quickly as possible in order to regale myself with a mug of beer in the cool of my veranda, this to recover from an unusually tough week. Before I could open my mouth, my visitor began to talk and continued to pour forth invective against the members of my profession, almost without pausing to take breath.

When he finally paused after twenty minutes of this I hastily said, "I'm very sorry but really there is nothing I can do to help you." For the first time he smiled broadly and replied, "But you have already helped me a great deal. You are the first person in three years who has bothered to listen to what I had to say. Thank you." Our positions were now reversed for he was in fact the "doctor" who first encouraged me to learn to listen. Now, some years later, I hope I can say that I have been a reasonably good pupil, one who has not disgraced his teacher.

Recently there have been reports that a number of cathedrals in the United Kingdom have set aside space as a "listening room." Members of the cathedral staff and other volunteers who help are trained not to counsel but to listen and give their time to all and sundry who need to unburden themselves of their problems, physical, mental, emotional, and spiritual. They then might ask what the person who came for help thinks is the answer to the problem. Counseling is something different, for which special arrangements have to be made.

———

Three of our "nudges," listening, caring, and praying, can often be combined into one. This is in fact the love of God, something much greater than purely human affection, such as liking someone or taking a fancy to a person, something that is the most powerful factor in the world. Physicists look for the "unifying force" that unites into one the forces of gravity, electromagnetic forces, and large and small nuclear forces. The Christian and the Jew believe they have found this unifying factor and call it love.

The attitudes of people who seek help from orthodox practitioners are changing. They are no longer prepared to take everything the doctor says as being gospel truth. They are prepared to listen, but they want then to be able to ask questions. And after that many of them want to make up their own minds as to whether they'll follow the doctor's advice or ask for another opinion, maybe from a practitioner of complementary medicine. If their doctor doesn't like that, they'll be prepared to get another doctor. The fact that this is beginning to happen already has had an effect on the physician in mainstream medicine. He or she is nowadays much more receptive to the idea of working with people who are practicing a different kind of medicine.

One of us was chatting a few weeks ago with a lady who had cancer. The oncologist had prescribed a course of chemotherapy. She agreed to this but asked advice from a number of friends. She decided to supplement chemotherapy with acupuncture and discovered the truth of what she'd been told, that the adverse effects of the chemotherapy were much less than expected. When asked if the oncologist knew she'd plumped for acupuncture she replied with a smile, " I really don't know. I never told him."

There is a problem here for patients who don't know much about taking care of themselves or about the things that make for a happy, healthy life. Some of these will be disturbed by the idea of having to stand up to the doctor and of making up their own minds. These people will need help. We hope that many physicians in all kinds of orthodox and complementary medicine will go out of their way to give help and advice to these people. There's a place for a new kind of doctor, one who makes it his or her concern to learn how to give patients advice and help them to find the therapist they need and with whom they'll feel comfortable, without imposing or leaning on them. The family doctor used to do this and sometimes still does. The nurse in the doctor's office may be the right person to do this now.

When the patient has said all he wants to get off his chest, the doctor has to decide how to respond. It may be right to ask one or two questions to clarify the situation. After that the best approach is to ask the patient what he thinks should be done. Two things are highly desirable. The first is to avoid laying down the law as to the treatment to be given; the second is to get the patient's cooperation in the plan of treatment. Many patients come because they want to be reassured. Often it's possible to give this reassurance and to do it with conviction.

In our orthopedic practice mothers often bring their young children, some worried that the kid's feet are turning in and others that they are turning out. In most instances one can reassure the anxious mother that there is no cause for anxiety, and that the apparent abnormality will correct itself quickly. In others it is necessary to supplement our opinion by prescribing a simple night splint, mainly to reassure the mother. In still others, a few, it is necessary to advise conservative or even operative treatment. The various possibilities have to be put to the parents in such a way as to get their agreement.

I (WHK-W) recall the case of a young schoolmaster with marked instability of the lower back at one level. We talked about this problem and I said, "Let's try simple measures first. You'll know for yourself if these give you sufficient help. Come back in three months. I hope that then you'll be free from pain. If not let's sit down together and think again." In three months he came back, still having quite severe back pain. We discussed this and agreed on a somewhat different approach. On the next visit he still had a lot of pain. I said, "It looks to me now that if the pain is severe enough we'll have to think about a bone-grafting operation to stabilize your back, but let's have one more go at another line of treatment, hoping to avoid the operation." He was happy to go along with this advice.

Three months later he came back and asked me to do the operation. Both of us felt good about the way we had tried to tackle this problem together. In hospital the night before operation I went to talk to him on the ward. I asked him if he had people in his church pray for him. He replied, "Do you think I'd let a man like you operate on my back without having the prayers of my friends at home!" I laughed at myself all the way back home. I prayed for him and for myself, too, for a successful operation. All went well, for me an easier operation than usual, for him less pain and a quicker convalescence than normal. At his last visit six months later, the bone grafts had taken, and he was free from pain. He said, "I must thank you, doctor, for all your help, but I have to tell you that I've bought a dog. I wanted to have someone I could kick around just as you have done to me!" We parted the best of friends.

After listening to the patient's satisfaction, the doctor gets into some discussion with the patient, asking questions and getting a response. The whole idea is to get the patient to take an active part in his or her own healing. Sometimes all the patient wants is reassurance that there's nothing serious wrong. The doctor's job is to reassure. A patient may be so worried that he or she can't listen to the doctor. Quite often when our patients go from the office to talk to the secretary about another appointment, they tell her that we never told them what was the matter. The secretary should do her part to reassure the patient. Even then the patient might tell the physical therapist, "No one told me what was wrong." So then we need to repeat the same message several times.

We were talking the other day about the schoolmaster who really needed an operation on his back but wasn't ready to accept it. The doctor played along for a year before the young man himself said he realized he needed an operation. It took time, but in the end the doctor-patient relationship was a right one. And we all know by now that the most important thing of all is the bond between patient and doctor. The patient talks; the doctor listens. Then they ask and answer questions, back and forth. At this point the doctor makes some tentative suggestions Her aim is always to get the patient to play a big role in his own treatment.

162

There's hell to pay when doctor and patient are not on the same wavelength. Occasionally one gets to hear a serious but amusing story. This one came years ago from friends telling us about their friends. An elderly couple both had cardiac problems, not serious ones, but the cardiologist sounded very serious. Neither husband nor wife could understand what the doctor said to them, at considerable length and in very complex language. A few weeks later both came back and the doctor, still incomprehensible, ordered a couple of tests on each of them, saying he couldn't tell them more till he got the results of the tests. They were depressed and so wandered off and drowned their sorrows in the rather pleasant pub on the wharf. That helped them to feel better, something more than the doctor had done.

Then the cardiologist went on vacation, without telling the patients the results of the tests. They rang his nurse, who said she couldn't possibly tell them the results; they'd have to wait till the doctor got back from his holiday in three weeks time. Down they went to the pub on the wharf and drowned their sorrows, and irritation, once again. This time they phoned the family doctor and told him it was getting rather expensive and could he put them in touch with a specialist who would show interest in helping them. He sent them to a very pleasant cardiologist who was on their wavelength and helped them quite quickly and simply to feel and to remain well again.

# − 19 −

# A Place to Linger

FOR THE PATIENT it is clearly more pleasant to be at home than in a hospital, unless he or she is seriously ill. Patients get well more quickly in a normal home environment. In a hospital it is much more difficult to avoid wounds and other infections. The costs of supporting patients in the hospital have escalated in recent years. This cost, so many tell us, will eventually become prohibitive. Some say that such costs will, before long, bankrupt the hospital.

For all these reasons it is highly advisable that the patient be treated at home, except when seriously ill or requiring complex postoperative care. We can envisage a shift to the small clinic for the treatment of most conditions, regardless of who the therapist may be. Anyone from aromatherapist to acupuncturist to orthoedic surgeon could be a part of this. This is the subject of the present discussion.

First, some general comments. What's to prevent the occurrence of disasters when orthodox and complementary forms of medicine stand side by side, and patients are free to choose the kind of treatment they prefer? One answer is that patients are not all that stupid and often know what they want and what they need as well or better than the physician does. Another answer is that physicians are not all that wise. Safeguards are readily available. If your patient is not improving, don't delay in arranging a second opinion. Except in emergencies the wise cardiac or spine surgeon seeks a consultation with the appropriate physician before embarking on any kind of operative intervention.

The same rule applies to those practicing in any branch of complementary medicine. Group practice in which different kinds of doctors work independently but in close contact is highly desirable. Frequent cross contacts in informal meetings are extremely helpful. It is said that Hippocrates and his colleagues and assistants used to meet every evening under the plane tree in their compound for wine and discussion of their patients' problems. His compound was a good example of a pleasant place near the sea in which to linger and get well again.

In recent years many corporations have designed their headquarters to impress the people who work inside them rather than to impress outsiders. British Airways has done this five miles west of London's Heathrow Airport. The main corridor that links several small office blocks is in fact a village street with grass and trees on either side of the lawns. The central buildings are designed to be like a village square. There is an underground car park, and those employed in the center have, on reaching street level, to walk across the village square to their offices, which are for the most part close to the areas in which those under them work. The bosses no longer work in areas isolated from the rest of the staff. This is a village in which people work hard in a very pleasant environment. The Canadian Telecoms company Nortel has moved its offices from central Toronto to a new self-contained small town in the suburbs with cafes, restaurants, indoor parks, and even a Zen garden. A big company outside Stockholm has its offices in a similar area, with indoor streets full of shops and cafes.

There are now several multidisciplinary clinics in North American cities, each with a variety of physicians of different kinds—family practitioners, orthopedic surgeons, physicians, radiologists, rheumatogists, psychologists, chiropractors, acupuncturists, physical and occupational therapists, and others—working individually and in close cooperation and interconnection when it's desirable to do so. We are not aware of any attempts to do this in a village atmosphere outside the city. We believe this to be highly desirable. As it is, these clinics from all accounts do a very good job and in the process both encourage one another and put the brakes on each other when necessary. The secret is frequent consultation and cross referral. The team's the thing.

We suggest that what remains to be done now is to transfer these activities to a rural village setting, one that is much more pleasant for both doctors, physicians, and patients. I (WHK-W) was fortunate thirty years ago in Nairobi to be responsible for orthopedic and rehabilitation work in a series of simply built offices, workshops, and wards arranged round a central garden. There were multicolored bougainvilleas and roses and, not the least important thing, an eighteen-hole golf course for hospital workers and others. For African patients coming from rural areas this was a very agreeable environment. It was almost a replica of their home environment. Much of the treatment was done in the open air. The patient's bed was often moved for part of each day into the garden. It was equally pleasant for surgeons, physical therapists, nurses, and others. Patients severely handicapped from poliomyelitis or from bone and joint tuberculosis made good recoveries under agreeable conditions. Eighty percent, at least, returned to active work again.

The foregoing suggests to us that the institution of an ideal setup in cities and, better still, in rural areas is now within our grasp both for patient and staff satisfaction and for cost effectiveness. Not far from the Pacific Rim city where one of us lives, there is a rural shopping center with a large market, constructed around a central square with room for parking cars. A hundred yards away, on a separate acre of land, is a chiropractor's office in an ideal situation with a view of the marina two hundred yards down the hill.

Such a setup, with help from entrepreneurs, could easily be developed to form the ideal grouping of small offices or of a rural multidisciplinary center. Another nearby small village has a shopping center with a pub, shopping center, family doctors' office, dentist, and physiotherapist's office, which could equally easily be developed to become an attractive center for similar multidisciplinary work.

In the city twenty miles away a sympathetic group of entrepreneurs, some of them physicians, could with some careful planning design the same sort of "little city" within a city, ideal for cooperation in medical work of a similar interdisciplinary nature. One acre adjoining a busy road in an industrial area of the city could, with planning, become a thriving center for complementary medical care, built around three sides of a square with a central grassy area shaded by pleasant trees. Half a mile away in a commercial shopping area the narrow streets lead down through a series of adjacent squares to the wharf and the harbor. These squares are surrounded by offices, greatly varying in style, all delightful. In one quiet corner is a small French restaurant, with tables outside on the square, managed by Breton people from the fishing town of Douarnenez in Brittany, people who showed great bravery in resisting the German invaders during the second World War. A judicious invasion of physicians of various kinds over a period of time could result in a most attractive medical center.

Appreciation of the value of an environment conducive to health is important; we need to pay much more attention to it. Looking back over three thousand years, we can read about similar attention to the healing environment, as was done in Delphi on Mount Parnassus at the Temple of Apollo, god of healing. Hippocrates worked in his small tree-shaded compound next to the harbor at Cos, a convenient location for many of his many patients who came from far away by sea.

Some years ago, looking for a place to have lunch in London, we stumbled on a small restaurant near a Chelsea square. We discovered that it was run by the people of the local Anglican church and, with a small adjacent bookstore, formed a welcome oasis in the midst of busy city streets. Because of the friendliness of those serving us, it achieved for tired, footsore people after a morning's shopping, what we've suggested for sick people needing help. We thought this was an excellent way for the church to make a weekday impact on those passing by without any unwelcome attempt to proselytize directly. Churches could well afford to do more of this, just as could physicians and those working with them. This kind of reaching out to strangers and welcoming of sick, tired people becomes automatically something extremely therapeutic.

# — 20 —

# Current Issues

D URING THE PAST DECADE, there has been a substantial increase, at least forty percent in the total number of visits to complementary and alternative medicine (CAM) providers in the North American continent. These visits actually exceed the total visits to all primary-care physicians, and it is estimated that several million adults take prescriptions concurrently with herbal remedies and/or high-dose vitamins. It is estimated that there is a low rate of disclosure by patients, regarding their use of CAM therapies, to their physicians. There is an increasing utilization of CAM therapies throughout the world.

A great deal of research into the utilization of CAM therapy has been accomplished, and, although the investigators would be too numerous to mention, some of the more prominent professionals would include Eisenberg, Pelletier, Haskell, Weil, Spiegel, Scholten, Rosenberg, Cherkin, Patton, and Cohen.

Many people pay out-of-pocket for their CAM therapy. A substantial percentage of people utilizing CAM therapy feel that the treatment was successful or that they were considerably improved. Frequently, visits for CAM therapy are for purposes of prevention or improvement in general health and not as much for treatment of disease. Studies have revealed that there is a tendency in people who utilize CAM therapy to have higher education levels, and their decisions for these types of services and products are based upon their concerns for their own health improvement.

In a great many instances, people seek out alternative therapy for chronic conditions, which include back problems and other chronically painful conditions, anxiety, depression, and other problems associated with mental health, headaches, allergies, upper respiratory tract infections, blood pressure, and GI problems. The most highly utilized therapies include acupuncture, chiropractic, energy healing, folk remedies, herbal medicine, homeopathy, massage, megavitamins, and various types of self-help groups. Many clinics and hospitals are offering many of these types of services, which also include holistic nursing, bodywork, biofeedback, guided imagery, hypnotherapy, nutrition, programs in women's health, and spiritual guidance, as well. Educational classes are becoming increasingly available at these medical centers.

Many people are satisfied with these types of therapies, and the success of such therapy, in many cases, may be at least in part based upon the belief that the therapy will work. The mindset of the patient can be a very powerful influence on the outcome of treatment. There appears to be a high satisfaction level among patients with acupuncture and chiropractic, and these therapies are utilized frequently as primary treatment.

There is evidence to show that a great many CAM therapy patients use these measures repeatedly and are not as concerned about unwanted side effects. However, the orthodox medical community feels that there are issues that need to be addressed, including safety, efficacy, cost effectiveness, and mechanisms of action in the individual alternative therapies. It appears that satisfactory research is lacking among many of these therapies, and there is an apparent lack of standardization, which would apply both to those that appear to be relatively safe and those that have demonstrated some degree of toxicity. Toxicities have been demonstrated with some herbal and vitamin supplements. There have been difficulties with conducting research for herbal products, as there is a lack of standardization of ingredients or dosage, and there may be more than one active ingredient present. There may be several components present in many traditional Chinese remedies.

There has been an increasing demand for evidence-based medicine over the past several years, with the advent of HMOs and managed care, as payers become increasingly concerned over the costs of health care. Many experts feel that the evaluation of CAM therapies might be best accomplished with randomized control trials. There has been relatively little support thus far from funding agencies for studies to investigate prevention.

The orthodox medical community is requesting more information regarding the potential risks and costs of therapy. Research is very costly and, therefore, certain therapies may be given priority over others in the evaluation process. As a prerequisite to such investigation, the appropriate treatment protocol would need to be selected by those therapists who utilize a particular methodology or technique. There have been randomized trials comparing chiropractic to physical therapy, and there have been some studies evaluating massage therapy and acupuncture as well. There is no evidence at this time to demonstrate that orthodox medicine is more effective for back pain than CAM therapies.

Orthodox and CAM therapists appear to agree that a vegetarian diet, in addition to various nutritional supplements, can make a contribution to the prevention of vascular disease, including heart attack and stroke and possibly some malignancies as well.

The current climate of health care would require not only that these alternative treatments be subjected to scientific testing for safety and efficacy, but that consumers be provided with acceptable factual information so they can make effective health care decisions, as the public is demonstrating an increasing interest in learning safe and effective treatment options for health care.

The orthodox health care community, in addition to insurance carriers and government regulatory agencies, have expressed interest in extending professional standardization to that sector of the CAM therapy community that might be lagging behind to some extent. There is now an express concern for improving the level of education and training, certification, and licensure of CAM health care professionals. There has been an increasing interest in including CAM into medical school curricula, residency training, continuing education, and faculty development, as well. Many feel at this time that there will need to be a coordination with many licensing organizations and the Federation of State Medical Boards.

Health plans will have a great deal to say regarding which therapies to cover and for which medical conditions, and they will also require the credentialing of providers. These agencies will develop cost-management strategies to monitor the quality of such treatment. While consumer preference is important, cost factors may eventually override such considerations.

It is of interest that at the present time there is a paucity of coverage for CAM therapies by insurance carriers, and there are significant limits on visits, in addition to relatively high copayments and deductibles. Insurance companies, in addition to placing a cap on covered benefits, are heading in the direction of requiring that such referrals be from an M.D. They are also dealing with the issue of providing these services for inpatients in hospitals. Coverage is currently being considered for certain medical problems including cancer, cardiovascular disease, musculoskeletal pain, and conditions concerning women's health.

Insurance companies and other payers are willing, in some measure, to meet the demands for CAM therapy, but other problems that confront them at this time include the attitude of many physicians and administrators, who have been reluctant to accept CAM therapies or, for that matter, many CAM practitioners as well. These problems are compounded by confusion regarding diagnostic and treatment coding, as the terminology among the orthodox and CAM therapy practitioners is not standardized. A final stumbling block in this process, as viewed by payers, is dealing with the belief systems regarding illness which are currently held by many CAM providers.

Government regulatory agencies will take an increasing role with respect to the utilization of CAM therapy, as they do with orthodox medicine, which would include scrutinizing unlicensed health care practice, deceptive advertising practices, any possible violations that may occur with controlled substances, and billing practices that may be considered fraudulent. There will be a continued careful approval process regarding drugs, foods, botanicals, biologics, medical devices, and labeling, as well as health and nutritional claims.

There will be legal issues that need to be carefully addressed, as liability will be related to credentialing and licensure, scope of practice, access to treatments or delayed access to treatments, professional disciplinary procedures, third-party reimbursement, in addition to health care fraud.

All of these issues are very real, and they must all be considered carefully as we move forward in the direction of integrating orthodox, complementary, and alternative medicine. There will need to be a proper balance achieved, with reasonable satisfaction to all parties involved, so that this direction of health care will benefit the public by an overall improvement in the public well-being.

# – 21 –

# Teaching and Learning

M OST THOUGHTFUL PEOPLE are aware that we are facing a crisis in the delivery of health care. Each group—physicians, payers, insurers, and others, patients, friends, and relatives—puts the responsibility for the crisis on others. More than anything else we need to understand that it is a symptom of a much larger problem, the need to teach medical students and others in all disciplines how to make decisions under conditions of uncertainty. At present we do not know how to do this, how to free our students from the pressure on them to accumulate an excessive number of facts and how to instill the practice of life-long scholarship. The problems that face medical schools of all disciplines today are far more than a question of unprecedented change and confusion. The opportunity for change to a far better system is a great one. To teach this in medical schools of all disciplines in a convincing way is a matter of vital importance.

It is helpful first to review two terms that are in common use today, epistemology and ontology. Epistemology deals with the study of the nature of knowledge, of what we actually can know in any given situation. Ontology describes reality, things as they really are, not just as we perceive them, a state of affairs seldom if ever arrived at in clinical practice. The eminent scientist and theologian John Polkinghorne reminds us that "epistemology models ontology," that what we are able to know in a particular situation is often a reliable guide to what is in fact the case. For us now this means that our striving for mutual understanding between the disciplines in health care has to take place in an atmosphere of uncertainty.

Wise men and women in the field of medicine in North America have made the point that we need to take a new look at both the teaching and learning of medical and postgraduate students in this time of crisis. This crisis is a combination of the effects of the information revolution, the cost-containment movement, the dissatisfaction of patients more alert than their predecessors, and the discontent of physicians and other health care deliverers in the loss of status. It is now essential to prepare students for medical practice under entirely new conditions.

These wise leaders in the education field believe that this tension is a symptom of a much larger problem, the conditions of uncertainty that are so prevalent in medical work, and which are even more cogent in the field of teaching. Some tell us that we do not know exactly what to teach and that it is important to free students from the need to amass an excessive number of facts and rather to teach the skills of life-long scholarship. One expert asks why we should give the members of the healing professions extraordinary rights and privileges at a time when their extraordinary knowledge is so much in question.

While discussing chaos theory in an earlier chapter, we saw that many events, including the Big Bang, took place under conditions of chaos, and that very small influences could be responsible for very marked changes, often leading to a state of greater order. We can be encouraged to think that in the uncertainty and chaos of our medical schools lies the germ of tremendous advance in the teaching and practice of health care and of preventive measures. Study of history shows that conditions of chaos have often led to changes that proved very beneficial to subsequent generations.

The American physician and teacher Dr. Donald Schon, summons us to a new approach that he calls "reflection-in-action." The process he advocates begins at the time when the patient enters the doctor's office, continues to the way the patient talks and behaves, and goes on to the making of a diagnosis and formulation of treatment. This often involves making judgments and employing skills for which one cannot explain the rules and procedures. The physician constantly questions what he observes during the history and physical examination, aiming to understand the patient as a whole person of body, mind, and spirit. Schon believes that this process of reflection-in-action is central to the practice of medicine.

Another American physician, Dr. Kent Bottles, has a number of suggestions to make in view of the foregoing. He proposes: (1) a medical school curriculum based on reflection-in-action; (2) concentration on the way in which competent physicians deal with the uncertainty of clinical practice; (3) teaching and learning by actually doing things, because (4) students can only educate themselves by embarking on doing things they do not at first understand. (5) The definition of health should be expanded to include the mental, social, and spiritual concerns that influence behavior and promote health. (6) The clinician must grasp the significance of the whole in order to understand any part of it.

The new approach suggested by Schon and Bottles calls for a reflection-in-action that focuses on the way in which the wise clinician deals with uncertainty, confusion, instability, uniqueness, and conflict of values. Chaos is compounded by the variety of different concepts of value held by those in many different disciplines today. At this stage in the development of relationships between one and another discipline in orthodox and complementary medicine, the most important quality is humility, that each one of us be aware that our ignorance is far greater than our knowledge. A practitioner in another discipline may have the answer to a problem that we find baffling.

We are reminded by "A Survey of the Twentieth Century" in the *Economist* of September 11, 1999, that "acceptance of a process of constant experimentation, involving the freely expressed views and actions of millions of people, is likely to produce a better, more adaptable outcome than one involving a committee of economists, politicians, bureaucrats, businessmen, or even journalists, drawing up a grand blueprint. This presumption is humble because is acknowledges the extent of our ignorance." As in economics, so in the teaching and practice of medicine of all disciplines.

Each contact of physician with patient calls for this kind of humility combined with marked sensitivity for the thoughts, feelings, and beliefs of the latter from start to finish. One begins the process by listening to the patient and then making very tentative suggestions in the hope that the patient himself will supply the answers for herself. As she then begins to ask us questions, we're in a position to make further comments, so that together we can reach the goal of health and healing for the individual and for society. A similar approach serves us well in the development of understanding between the members of the various disciplines.

It's one thing to list and discuss the problems, or as business manager Roger Ackhoff would say, the messes. To come to a conclusion about making the right solutions is quite a different matter. At the beginning of this book we talked about the "togetherness" of people and things according to Bell's Theorem in our quantum world. It is more than likely that the answers we seek will become apparent as we get together to discuss the problems that face us, and we should do this in a way that we find as interesting and as enjoyable as possible.

From consideration of things discussed in earlier chapters, it becomes clear that two matters are of extreme importance: (1) a thorough and complete diagnosis and (2) emphasis on the importance of education. The common practice in the past when faced with a problem has been to call a committee or set up a commission. There are some people who love committees and a few who feel they are pulling their weight only when sitting in a committee meeting. Most of us find committees extremely boring. We believe that the meeting of minds to solve a problem should be informal and enjoyable. The main achievement of the American Back Society has been to get people of very diverse interests in the healing professions together in the most informal way possible.

In this society the more formal sessions to read and to listen to short presentations on a variety of topics have been important. The information gained has been useful in promoting mutual understanding between people in diverse disciplines. Even more important have been the times spent together outside of formal sessions. Exchanges over a mug of ale or a glass of wine or at lunch or dinner have been very effective. To discover common interests outside of professional concerns does much to overcome prejudices between people that often have an emotional rather than a logical foundation. When two or three people discover over dinner that they are enthusiasts of impressionist painting or golf or scuba diving, the fact that one is a chiropractor, another a naturopath, and another an orthopedic surgeon pales into insignificance.

The American Back Society has in our opinion done more than any other body in these respects. The members look forward to meeting one another as old friends each year and pursuing common interests much more than acquiring new knowledge or honing new skills. We come to know each other as individuals with many common human interests, and this lays the basis for working together as health care professionals.

It is important to have small meetings of professionals on frequent occasions. The colleges at Oxford and Cambridge have been unique in this respect. Their methods fortunately have now been adopted in many universities throughout the world. In these British universities each of a number of colleges has its quota of fellows, classical scholars, scientists, historians, sociologists, and others, who teach and do research in various departments and dine together in the college hall, relaxing together in the senior common room over port afterwards, several times each week. Friendships are cemented, legs are pulled, projects and deep interests are discussed, and the first steps are taken in planning work that not infrequently leads to a Nobel Prize.

A similar approach is taken by the staff of the Campbell Clinic in Memphis, Tennessee. On one evening each week the staff and residents meet to discuss treatment given to individual patients during the previous week. Following this there is time for staff members or residents to raise for discussion any matter of importance to them. The voicing of a grievance or a simple suggestion is in this setting of great value in that each person, junior or senior, comes to feel that he or she can participate in the running of the clinic.

When we do get together to solve a problem or clear up a mess, in whatever walk of life it may be, it is wise to start quietly and slowly, taking time to assess the nature of the problem. If there are difficulties, it may be wise to adjourn the meeting and to come together for further discussion in a few days time. Quite often, as a group of people discusses a problem, the solution gradually becomes apparent without any conscious attempt to do so. It is a fatal mistake to rush to the solution without due consideration of all the aspects involved. The wise chairman or member is one who is prepared to listen rather than force his or her opinion. The really valuable member of the group is the man or woman who is prepared to admit to being ignorant or inadequate, looking to others for enlightenment.

It pays to appear humble even when one does not feel that way! When the nature of the problem has been made clear, it is sensible to ask pertinent questions rather than give a forceful opinion off the cuff. Time taken to understand fully the viewpoint of others is time well spent. Two members of a committee in which no agreement has been reached may suddenly arrive at a solution while playing golf or sitting on the patio having a beer, not thinking of that problem at all. The solution suddenly comes.

In the first chapter while discussing chaos theory we concluded that small changes at the start of a process or reaction often lead to large changes at the end. We listed the little ripples that had a deleterious effect on a patient's progress and the little nudges that led to marked improvement. Similar ripples and nudges are effective in a many different situations, such as learning to understand the thought processes of a health care professional in a different discipline, something we all have to tackle nowadays. We suggest that the reader refer back to the Chapter Two to remind yourself of these ripples and nudges, which are such powerful tools and so readily available to us at a very small cost.

At the beginning of this chapter we stressed the vital importance of two different aspects of our problem, diagnosis and education. We remind ourselves that making a complete and thorough diagnosis includes not only the physical condition of the patient but also his or her mental state, beliefs, likes and dislikes, conditions at home and at work, and the way he or she interacts with other people. This interaction includes physicians and other professionals, nurses, insurers, and others. To make an adequate diagnosis may be a very simple matter, as in treating a minor injury in a happy and healthy person, or it may be extremely complex, calling for help from a number of different specialists. Much suffering and expense can be avoided by the early recognition of a complicated problem. In cases where there is not marked improvement or where there is delay in helping the patient back to work, it is essential to obtain the help of those working together in a multidisciplinary clinic or other similar institution.

In this book we have tried to deal with some of the problems that affect people of many different disciplines in orthodox and in complementary medicine. In this chapter we have discussed some of the things that are of great importance in promoting cooperation between people in different disciplines. This is where emphasis on education is so important. Our task is not only to educate ourselves and one another but to initiate this process in our students. The word "education" comes from two Latin words that imply a "leading forth." It is up to us to lead one another on to the place of mutual understanding. We are still learning how to interact with other professionals. The criteria involved in assessing outcomes and in setting up controlled double-blind studies are still not yet well delineated. How then can we set about the very difficult task of educating our students in the midst of so much uncertainty ?

We have considered briefly a number of possible procedures. Past experience can help us; intuition is often called for. We are all traveling together along an unknown path to an equally unknown destination. Christopher Columbus did this, with results that changed the world. For all of us this could be an exciting, enjoyable experience, and the end results could be abundantly rewarding.

# — 22 —

# Thrusting Through the Waves

I (WHK-W) GREW UP in a home on the Kentish cliffs seven miles north of Dover. I was fascinated by the ships, trawlers, tankers, container ships, and liners taking passengers to India, Australia, and the Far East. My coauthor (AAS) has lived and worked near the San Francisco Bay. He too has the sea and all its excitements in his blood. There's nothing more exciting than to watch a ship thrusting through the waves on her way to discharge her pilot at Dover or speeding majestically beneath the Golden Gate Bridge.

Health care is like a ship thrusting its way ahead boldly through the waves created by turbulent conditions in our modern world, carrying us to an exciting but unknown destination. First our forebears and now we, ourselves, have witnessed many changes in the way health care has been delivered. We've talked briefly about the origins of modern medicine in Chinese, Grecian, and Judeo-Christian culture. The rate of change has been greater than ever since the time of the American Civil War in the 1860s. In his book *Healing Words*, Dr. Larry Dossey has outlined the three modern eras:

Era I had local, Newtonian physical medicine dominating the field, described in terms of space-time-matter-energy, where the mind is an example of a brain mechanism. Most forms of modern medicine and drugs, surgery, irradiation, and chemotherapy fall into Era I. From the middle of the eighteenth century till 1940 more attention was given to the importance of the physical than to the mental aspects of disease. The mind was synonymous to the brain, localized within the cranium in space and in time.

Era II is described as local mind-body medicine. From 1940 on, mind came to be regarded as a major causal factor, not fully explained by classical physical concepts. Examples are biofeedback, relaxation, and imagery. Mind was thought to be localized to the individual in space and time.

Era III is nonlocal. Mind is not completely localized in space or in time, whether conscious or unconscious. From 1980 on, medicine cannot be described by classical concepts of space-time-matter-energy. Examples are diagnosis and healing at a distance, telesomatic events, prayer, and therapeutic touch.

Over the years the ship has steamed from the home waters, where all the emphasis was on physical. clock-like concerns, well-defined and localized, to the open sea, where much more emphasis is placed on the way the mind affects the body, but always within the one single person. Now our vessel is traveling in oceans where the seas are more boisterous and the wind blows a gale. The mind still controls the physical body, but it is no longer considered purely local in space or in time. Its action is no longer limited to one individual. There is a spread of "mind" from person to person, involving groups of people. This is particularly obvious in considering the unconscious mind, where the spread is far greater than we can imagine. Carl Jung talked about the "collective unconscious," where all are one. According to this concept, health is no longer an individual affair. All people are interrelated and interdependent, the well-being of one affecting others.

It was said of Harold Wilson, Britain's prime minister in the 1950s, that like Christopher Columbus, as he started his voyage he did not know where he was going, when he got to the far country he did not know where he was, and when he got back home he did not know where he had been.

We can modify this statement to explain our own situation. We know the place from which we set out on our voyage to the Fair Health Country; we have a good idea of where we are now. We have only the haziest idea of whither we are traveling or what the unseen country will be like. We can guess that all the disciplines in medicine will turn out to be interconnected, each one an integral part of the whole, that we physicians will be one with each other and with our patients. We envision that the pursuit of health will be something positive and pleasant, freed from the fear and uncertainty of the present struggle to eradicate disease, as our ship thrusts forward confidently through the waves, carrying us to the land where the inhabitants are bursting with health.

The nonlocal nature of mind can be seen in the experiments of the Princeton University Engineering Anomalies Research Group. In one set of these experiments trained researchers sent "thought messages" of several pages to other similarly trained researchers in a country such as Singapore, on the other side of the world. These latter received ninety percent of each message correctly. One aspect of the experiments was totally unexpected: some of the messages were apparently received three days before they were sent! These and other similar experiments demonstrate that mind is nonlocal, not only in space but in time as well.

Proponents of the new physics tell us that "epistemology models ontology": what we can and do know is a reasonable guide to the way things actually are. From what we know at present we can make some reasonable guesses for the future. The new approach to health will call for wide review, so that all disciplines have more knowledge about the things that are offered by each other and the way they are put into practice. It will demand the allocation of more time in medical and postgraduate school for study and observation of the work of many disciplines other than one's own and the institution of refresher courses for those already qualified. These studies will need to put much more emphasis on practical work, visiting other treatment centers, learning at first hand how one and another discipline conduct their practices and how they may best cooperate with each other.

There is clear evidence of the benefits to be obtained from an agreeable environment where different disciplines can work in close proximity, even in an urban setting but preferably in a rural one. To encourage the building and staffing of such centers is to take one of the most effective steps forward.

Looking ahead to the future in the midst of a busy professional life demands a great deal from every one of us, but it is something that will pay big dividends. The setting up of a number of small groups of ten to twelve members from the different disciplines in as many different areas as possible to discuss possible future changes could pave the way for action in the future. It isn't good enough to wait until the need for change suddenly becomes obvious, so that drastic changes are made without due deliberation. As acupuncturists, aromatherapists, chiropractors, herbal therapists, homeopaths, massage therapists, naturopaths, orthodox physicians, osteopaths, physical therapists, therapeutic massage therapists, and others get used to one another and learn to discuss health problems together, we can expect a great deal of valuable new insight into one another's problems and, even more important, into those of our patients. This is naturally best done in the pleasant informal atmosphere of a home, garden, or country club.

From the knowledge we have gained of many different disciplines and from discussion with colleagues, both in our own area and in others, we have little doubt that each discipline needs to review the contents of its syllabus with comprehensive change in mind. There is far too much emphasis on detail and not nearly enough on overall principles. Of course it is not possible to lay down effective principles without recourse to facts, but there is little to be gained by cluttering the mind with a plethora of detail when the facts can be looked up in the appropriate textbook with ease. We've already referred to Einstein's approach to this.

We recall the case of the lecturer with a Ph.D. in microbiology who moved from Europe to America to teach in a university department . He had to pass an entrance examination to allow him to practice in the state where he was going to work. He failed one part of the exam, microbiology, because he couldn't remember which bacteria were lactose fermenters! This was the kind of thing he'd look up when necessary. Years ago I (WHK-W) had to sit for an examination in one of the states in North America. The examination in medical jurisprudence consisted of the translation of a dozen legal terms from Latin to English. Some knowledge of Latin gave me a pass mark. Was this exam important, or was it designed to enable the examining board to fail applicants according to their whims and fancies?

Physicians of the bleeding-purging-cupping age would no doubt be overwhelmed with confusion were they to come back to Earth today to be confronted with the completely changed outlook in medical care. Change takes place in every sphere of human action now with an unheard-of degree of speed. It is almost certain that were those of us in medicine at the present time to come back to Earth in a hundred years, we'd be equally flummoxed. Even in ten or fifteen years the state of medical practice will almost certainly be unrecognizable by today's standards.

With all this in mind, it is worthwhile to take the risk of making what might at first sight appear to be a preposterous suggestion. We would advocate changing medical education to one fundamental curriculum embracing every discipline. The first three years would be study of basic subjects common to all disciplines. At end of these years the decision would be made by each individual as to which discipline he or she would chose to practice. The three final years of study would be in the chosen field, be it chiropractic, osteopathic, naturopathic, homeopathic, orthodox medicine, preventive medicine, public health, or other. On qualification, one year would be required as an intern in the chosen discipline, during which there would be contacts between disciplines. In the case of internal medicine, surgery, psychiatry, and similar very specialized subjects, further study would of course be necessary, again varying in length and content from one subject to another.

Our ship has traveled far from the port of departure to a new and foreign land. But it's a very exciting land. No doubt when we get there we'll be tackling new problems and seizing new opportunities.

# — 23 —

# Tomorrow's World

IN CHAPTER TWO we began to think about the nature of the world in which we live and work, through the medium of Newtonian and quantum physics. As we've journeyed together we've learned that there are more ways than one of looking at a problem: that patient, wife or husband, relatives, friends, nurses, and doctors of all sorts are so very closely connected that they affect one another; that the attitude of the doctor has an enormous effect on the health of the patient; and that what we call "mind" and what we call "body" are not two separate things but a combination that forms one entity. In a sense mind is the pattern, the real self, that is expressed while we're on this earth through our bodies. Reminding ourselves of Bell's Theorem, we can appreciate that minds, like subatomic particles, are non-local, not subject to the limitations of space or time. It follows that what we call "prayer" is not just words but an attitude, a feeling of something more than good will, that speeds from one person or persons to another, regardless of distance.

On several occasions we've discussed the influence for healing that a whole list of "little nudges" has on a patient's recovery. Each of the items on the list tells us of a way of transferring information from physician to patient. At the bottom of the list is the most important item—

prayer, an activity that is grossly underestimated and equally misunderstood. One small girl of four or five years old after church one Sunday sat on her grandfather's knee and suddenly asked him, "Grandpa why is prayer so noisy?" Fortunately grandpa remembered the story of another small girl of thirteen or so who, sitting on her grandfather's knee asked, "Grandpa, if you want to pray for someone who is sick, how do you do it?" "You just take him or her into your heart and lift your friend up into God's loving arms," came the answer. Then the first grandfather was able to tell his granddaughter that prayer didn't have to be noisy.

A report in a recent number of the *Mayo Clinic Women's Health Source* recognizes prayer as an important complementary medical treatment and states that, while in the nineteenth and twentieth centuries faith was taken out of the spotlight and replaced with modern medicine, today more than thirty medical schools in the U.S., including the Mayo Clinic, teach courses on spirituality and religion, up from just three schools three years ago.

Recent surveys show that seventy-five percent of patients in the U.S. believe that their physician should address spiritual issues with them and that fifty percent would like their doctor to pray with or for them. Many physicians do pray quietly for their patients. A distinguished eye surgeon in western Canada asks his patients if they would like him to pray with them before he starts an operation. I (WHK-W.) found that if I and the patient prayed before an operation, the whole procedure went more smoothly than usual, there was less pain after the surgery, and the recovery was speedier.

There have been over 130 scientific controlled studies on the effects of the equivalent of prayer—thoughts directed for the well-being of the subject at a distance—whether human being, plant, bacterium, or other object. In fifty percent of these the findings strongly suggest that prayer has been at work. (See Larry Dossey's book *Healing Words*).

Many distinguished scientists have believed in the existence of God, a creator and supreme being who is beyond and above personality. Einstein said that one of the chief reasons for his work was to discover more of the nature of God. Max Planck, one of the founders of quantum theory, had similar beliefs. Paul Davies, the popular scientific writer, wrote that he thought that science was a surer way to God than religion.

It's natural to ask "But what sort of a God? Did God set the clock ticking, as Newton believed, and then leave it to itself? Did God so arrange the foundation of the universe and so organize things that from there on it could make itself, and our world in it, step by step over fifteen billion years? And still more important, does God continue to have an interest in our universe, in our world and its people and in their well being?"

A hint of the answer comes in the true story of a German concentration camp during World War II. For no reason other than brutality, young Stephan, a Jewish lad of seventeen, was strung up to be hanged. Nearby Jewish prisoners were compelled to watch this. As the boy twisted and struggled after the rope was tightened, several of them grunted, "And where is our God now?" The answer came from one of them, "He's there with Stephan in the noose." During the terrible brutalities in Kosova, in East Timor, and in Chechnya, the answer to the question "Where is God now?" is the same. God is there with all suffering people. Many of us believe that God is near and caring for all of creation and that our prayers are powerful thoughts of love and well-being for those in need.

It is important for all of us to recognize the "little nudges" we have talked about so often as the equivalent of prayer. John Polkinghorne has helpful ideas about this. Our universe, writes this learned man, often exhibits twin processes. The impetus of the Big Bang drives the galaxies apart, while the pull of gravity works to pull them together. In it there are factors described by Newton that are "clocklike" as well as others, mentioned by modern scientists, that are quantum, "cloud like." Many phenomena in our world are surrounded by uncertainty. This gives God some room to maneuver. His nature is Newtonian on the one hand, in that he can't break his own rules. At the same time God has to give himself the freedom to react to the nudge, a big nudge perhaps, that comes to him through prayer and makes him a personal God.

In our prayer nudges we need some room to maneuver. To think of laser light helps us to grasp something of the efficacy of many people praying together for one or another person or state of affairs. Laser light is coherent light of which the waves are all in step and thus so much more powerful. Laser light can weld two sheets of metal together or bore a hole through a diamond. Laser prayer is equally powerful. A Roman writer once said, *Laborare est orare*, to work is to pray.

One of us lives on Vancouver Island and looks out of the study window at the spring flowers and shrubs in the garden, crocuses, daffodils, tulips, multicolored anemones, and forsythia, with a strip of the Pacific Ocean and the blue hills of Washington State in the distance beyond. In the eye of the mind he can picture the blossoms on the fruit trees soon to come. The other one, living in California, also near the sea, can delight in roses of many shades, bougainvilleas, geraniums, and snapdragons, with jacarandas soon to flower and the masses of purple status soon to color the hillsides. This makes it easy for us to envisage the future garden of health care, which itself is multicolored in its splendor, with blossoming professionals of all kinds within its sphere.

# About the Authors

DR. WILLIAM H. KIRKALDY-WILLIS (M.D., LL.D., F.R.C.S., F.A.C.S., F.I.C.C.) was educated at Cambridge and London in the 1930s, and spent the early years of his medical career in Africa, mostly in Kenya, before moving to Canada. He is Emeritus Professor and head of the Department of Orthopedic Surgery, University of Saskatchewan College of Medicine, and the former Senior Surgical Specialist to the Government of Kenya.

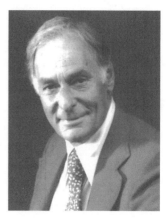

AUBREY SWARTZ (M.D., Pharm.D.) received his pharmaceutical doctorate at The University of Southern California, his Doctor of Medicine degree at UC Irvine School of Medicine, and trained in Orthopedic surgery at the University of Miami Medical Center. He has been in private preactice for many years and has been a clinical instructor and assistant professor at UCSF Department of Orthopedic Surgery. In 1982, Dr. Swartz founded the American Back Society.

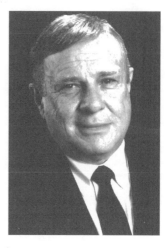

# Index

## A

ABS. *See* American Back Society
Ackhoff, Roger, 138–39, 180
acupressure, 85
acupuncture, 82, 85–86, 172
Aesculapius, 4, 6
Africa, 40–41, 51–53, 77, 167
Aix-les Bains, France, 91
American Back Society (ABS), 6,
    17–21, 40, 180–81
American Medical Association
    (AMA), 27–28, 31, 45, 64–65
anesthetics, 26
antibiotics, 30–31, 36–37
antibodies, 117
Apollo, 1, 2, 6, 141, 149, 168
appendicitis, 29, 73
aromatherapy, 99–102
asking, importance of, 157, 160, 161,
    162
aspirin, 30, 84
asthma, 48, 62
atherosclerosis, 105
autonomic nervous system, 109
ayurvedic medicine, 103–4, 110

## B

back pain, 137–38. *See also* American
    Back Society
bacteria, 116
Bailey, Hamilton, 33
Bastyr University, 95–96
Bath, England, 91
B-cells, 117
Bell, John, 12

Bell's Theorem, 9, 12, 13, 128–29,
    180, 191
Benson, Herbert, 110, 111
Berck Plage, France, 92
biofeedback, 109, 186
Blanchard, K., 139
Bohr, Nils, 13
bonuses, 143
Bothel, Washington, 95
Bottles, Kent, 179
bras, 129–30
breast cancer, 29, 129–30
British Airways, 166

## C

Cameron, Ewan, 125
Campbell Clinic, 142, 181–82
Canadian College of Naturopathic
    Medicine, 96
Canadian Memorial Chiropractic
    College, 5–6, 54
cancer, 123–31
    books on, 130–31
    breast, 29, 129–30
    guided imagery and, 109–10
    interconnectedness and, 128–29
    naturopathy and, 94–95
    nonmedical problems associated
        with, 128
    other factors in, 129–30
    remission of, 124
    stress and, 130
    testicular, 130
    treatment of, 124–26
Cannell, Winifred, 78

CEOs, role of, 138–41
cervical spine therapy, 57
chaos theory, 7, 14–15, 95, 178, 182
chelation, 105
China, 1, 25, 81, 111. *See also*
    Traditional Chinese Medicine
chiropractic, 51–65
    acceptance of, 56, 65
    cooperation between orthodox
        medicine and, 54–56, 59–62
    criticism of, 62
    current practice of, 56–57, 58–59,
        147
    effects of, 56–57
    experiences with, 51–53
    history of, 63–65
    physical therapy vs., 75
    rivalry between orthodox medicine
        and, 28
    satisfaction with, 172
Clarke, Andrew, 146
clocks, 10, 14, 193
clouds, 10, 14, 193
colonic lavage, 97
Columbia Advanced Practice Nurse
    Association, 152
complementarity, 11
complementary medicine. *See also*
    *individual therapies*
    areas done well, 39
    areas needing improvement, 39
    conditions treated by, 172
    evaluation of, 173
    governmental regulation of, 174–75
    increased utilization of, 171
    insurance and, 174
    legal issues and, 175
    most highly utilized, 172
    orthodox medicine's view of,
        172–74
    satisfaction with, 171–72
complement cascade, 120
computer use, 59
conventional medicine. *See* orthodox
    medicine
convents, 149
Corinth, 76, 149
Cos, 1, 4, 6, 20, 25, 68, 76, 168
counseling, 159
Cousins, Norman, 129
Cowden, Lee, 130
craniosacral therapy, 57, 58, 70
Creighton, James, 130

**D**

Davenport, Iowa, 63, 69
Davies, Paul, 15, 193
Delpech, Jacques, 76–77
Delphi, 1–4, 6, 20, 149, 168
Descartes, Rene, 12
detoxification, 47, 97, 104
Diamond, John, 130
digitalis, 30
Divine Ploughman, 87
doctors
    importance of listening and asking
        for, 157–63, 180
    interaction between patients and,
        58, 126–27, 157–63, 180, 192
    patients' selection of, 49
Dossey, Larry, 107, 185, 192
Droitwich, England, 91
drugs, 30–31
Dupytren, Dr., 33

**E**

EDTA, 105
Edward VI, 29
Einstein, Albert, 10, 188, 193
electromagnetism, 106
elements, five, 87
Epidauros, 1, 4, 20, 149
epistemology, 177–78, 187
essential oils, 99–100

**F**

Feinstein, Alice, 130
Fitzgerald, William, 111
Fleming, Alexander, 30, 36
Flexner, Abraham, 31
Florey, Howard Walter, 30, 36
food supplements, 119–20

**G**

Gattefosse, Rene-Maurice, 100
Gerber, Richard, 107
God, 192–93
Goldberg, Burton, 130–31
Graham, Sylvester, 27
gravity, 106
Greece, ancient, 1–5, 20, 76, 141,
    149
Greenman, Philip, 69, 70
Grenfell, Wilfred, 29
group practice. *See* multidisciplinary
    clinics
Guild of Barber Surgeons, 25

**H**

Hadler, Nortin, 138, 145, 147
Hahnemann, Samuel, 26, 43–44, 46
Hahnemann Hospital, 45
Hall, Justice, 5
Halstead, Dr., 29
Harrison, Edward, 68

Harvard University Medical School,
    31
healing centers, ancient, 1–5, 20. *See
    also* multidisciplinary clinics
Heisenberg's Uncertainty Principle,
    11, 13
Henry VIII, 150
Heracles, 4, 6
herbal medicine, 86–90
Hippocrates, 4–5, 6, 25, 44, 68, 76,
    91, 141, 166, 168
Hippocratic Oath, 5
Holmes, Oliver Wendell, 68
home
    influence of, 133–36
    treatment at, 165
homeopathy, 43–50
    cooperation between orthodox
        medicine and, 48–50
    criticisms of, 46, 48
    current practice of, 47, 49
    history of, 26, 43–47
    popularity of, 43
    studies of, 48
Hopkins, Gowland, 120
Huang Di, 87
Hunt, Agnes, 78

**I**

imagery, guided, 109–10
immune system, 115–21
    functioning of, 116–18
    importance of, 115–16
    maintaining health of, 119–21, 125
immunization, 27, 35
indeterminacy, 10–11
infinitesimals, law of, 44
Ingham, Eunice, 111–12
insurance, 174

interdisciplinary clinics. *See* multidisciplinary clinics

**J**

James, Dr., 146
Japan, 81, 147
Jenner, William, 27, 46
Johnson, S., 139
Jones, Robert, 68, 78
Jung, Carl, 186

**K**

Keer Keer, Frank, 77–78
Kennedy, John, 72
Kneipp, Sebastian, 91

**L**

Lane, Arbuthnot, 29
laughter, 129
leucocytes, 116
lifestyle, healthy, 121
Lincoln, Abraham, 45
listening, 157–63
Lister, Joseph, 26
Liverpool, 68
Love, Robert McNeill, 33
Lown, Bernard, 157–58
Lubcke, Dr., 147
Luckes, Miss, 154–55
Lust, Benedict, 91
Luton, England, 145
lymphocytes, 116–17

**M**

macrophages, 116
magnetic therapy, 106–8
Maimonides, 99
mainstream medicine. *See* orthodox
medicine

mantra, 111
manual medicine, 70, 71, 72
Margate, England, 92
marriage, 134–36
Mayo Clinic, 28–29, 139, 141, 192
medical education
medieval, 25
in the first half of the 20th century,
31–35
today, 40, 177–78, 179, 192
future, 189
meditation, 110–11
Memphis, Tennessee, 142, 181
meridians, 82–84, 85–86
Michaud, Ellen, 130
Mierau, Dale, 54, 56, 144–45, 147
mind and body, 12–13, 185–87, 191
mind-body therapy, 108–11
mobilization, 75
Molony, David, 87
monasteries, 25, 149–50
"mouse syndrome," 59
moxibustion, 85
multidisciplinary clinics, 61–62, 147,
166–69, 183, 188

**N**

Nairobi, Kenya, 51–53, 77, 167
National College, 95
naturopathy, 91–98
colleges for, 95–97
cooperation between orthodox
medicine and, 94, 97–98
criticism of, 97
current practice of, 94–95
history of, 91–93
popularity of, 92–93
principles of, 91, 93–94
Newton, Isaac, 8, 193

New York, 151, 152
Nightingale, Florence, 150
Nortel, 166
nudges, 7–8, 14–15, 49, 129, 182,
   191–92
Nugent, John, 64
nursing, 149–55
  history of, 149–51
  recent trends in, 152, 153–54
  training for, 151–52

## O

observer and observed, linkage of,
   11–12, 57–58
Oklahoma City, Oklahoma, 69
ontology, 177–78, 187
orthodox medicine. *See also* medical
  education
  areas done well, 38
  areas needing improvement, 38
  cooperation between complementa-
    ry medicine and, 38–40
  history of, 25–29, 35–37, 185–86
Osler, William, 68
osteopathy, 67–74
  cooperation between orthodox
    medicine and, 28, 72, 74
  current practice of, 71
  experiences with, 71–72, 73
  history of, 26, 67–71
  physical therapy vs., 75
  rivalry between orthodox medicine
    and, 28, 70–71
  studies of, 72–73
Oswestry, England, 77, 78

## P

Paget, James, 68
Palmer, B. J., 63–64

Palmer, D. D., 63, 65, 69
Paracelsus, 44
Pasteur, Louis, 26
patients
  doctor selection by, 49
  importance of attitude of, 94–95,
    172
  interaction between doctors and,
    58, 126–27, 157–63, 180, 192
Pauling, Linus, 119, 120, 125, 130
Peale, Norman Vincent, 119
Penfield, Wilder, 141
penicillin, 30, 36
Pergamum, 1
Perkins, George, 78
Peters, Ellis, 150
phagocytic cells, 116
pharmaceutical companies, 31
physical therapy, 75–80
  chiropractic vs., 75
  cooperation between orthodox
    medicine and, 77–78, 80
  current practice of, 75, 78–80
  experiences with, 77–78
  history of, 76–77
physicians. *See* doctors
physics, 7, 8–15
physiotherapy, 77
Planck, Max, 10, 193
Plewes, Dr., 145
Polkinghorne, John, 15, 93, 178, 193
Popular Health Movement, 27
Portland, Oregon, 95
positive thinking, 119
Potter, Gordon, 5, 54
prana, 103
prayer, 111, 160, 162, 186, 191–94
Princeton University Engineering
    Anomalies Research Group, 187

Prontosil, 36
psychoneuroimmunology, 108, 131
pulses, 84–85

**Q**

quantum physics, 7, 8–15
qi, 82–84, 103

**R**

reflection-in-action, 178–79
reflexology, 111–12
relationships, 134–36
relaxation, 110–11, 186
religion, 93–94, 149, 160. *See also*
    God; prayer; spiritual issues
reticulo-endothelial system, 115
Reynaud's syndrome, 109
ripples, 7, 14–15, 182
Robbins, John, 127, 130
Rochester, Minnesota, 28, 139
Rosenfeld, Isadore, 87, 130

**S**

salary, 142–43
salicylic acid. See aspirin
Sandoz, Dr., 56
Saskatoon, Saskatchewan, 54, 142
Schon, Donald, 178–79
self-employment, 138
Semmelweiss, Ignaz, 26
Seward, William Henry, 45
sex, 76, 134, 149
Shealy, Norman, 107
Sheng Yang, 87
Siegel, Bernie, 130
similars, law of, 44
Simonton, Stephanie and Carl, 130
Simpson, James, 26

Southwest College of Naturopathic
    Medicine, 96
spas, 91–92
spiritual issues, 192. *See also* God;
    prayer; religion
Still, Andrew, 26, 63, 68–70, 74
streptomycin, 30, 36
stress, 111, 130
succussion, 44
sulphonamides, 30, 36
Sutherland, Donald, 54
Swartz, Aubrey and Nedra, 17, 18, 20
Swedish massage, 77
Sydney, Australia, 77

**T**

T-cells, 117–18
teaching, 177–78, 179
Tempe, Arizona, 95, 96
testis, cancer of, 130
therapeutic touch, 111, 186
Thomas, Hugh Owen, 67–68
Thomson, Samuel, 27
Toronto, Ontario, 95, 96
Traditional Chinese Medicine (TCM),
    81–90. *See also* acupuncture;
    herbal medicine
  characteristics of, 81–82
  cooperation between orthodox
    medicine and, 82
  principles of, 82–85, 87
Transcendental Meditation, 110
Travell, Janet, 72
Treves, Frederick, 29
turbulence, 15

**U**

uncertainty, 11

## V

Valnet, Jean, 100
Vear, Herbert, 54
vertebral artery, 60–61
viruses, 116, 117–18
visualization, 120–21
vitamin supplements, 119–20, 125

## W

Wedge, John, 5
Weil, Andrew, 87
Wilson, Harold, 186
work disability, 146
workplace, 137–48
    back pain related to, 137–38
    CEO's role, 138–41
    importance of ambience of,
        138–42, 147
    salaries and bonuses, 142–43
    subordinate managers' role,
        143–44
    visits to, 144–48, 154
World Health Organization, 48, 50

## Y

Yellow Emperor, 87
yin and yang, 82–84, 85, 87
yoga, 110

## Z

Zen Buddhism, 110
Zukav, Gary, 15